Care Staff Mobilisation i

Ivan Sainsaulieu

# Care Staff Mobilisation in the Hospital

Fight or Cooperate?

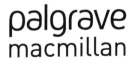

Ivan Sainsaulieu
University of Lille
Lille, France

ISBN 978-981-19-9353-4          ISBN 978-981-19-9354-1   (eBook)
https://doi.org/10.1007/978-981-19-9354-1

Cover pattern © Melisa Hasan

This Palgrave Macmillan imprint is published by the registered company Springer Nature Singapore Pte Ltd.
The registered company address is: 152 Beach Road, #21-01/04 Gateway East, Singapore 189721, Singapore

*To my daughter Nina, hoping that she will be able to benefit from quality public hospitals ... or that she will be able to fight for it.*

# Acknowledgements

Many thanks to the nurses and healthcare workers who took care of this book by agreeing to meet me to discuss about it.

Thanks to the University of Lille and Clersé laboratory for having accepted to financially support this book.

Thank you Muriel, for putting up with me.

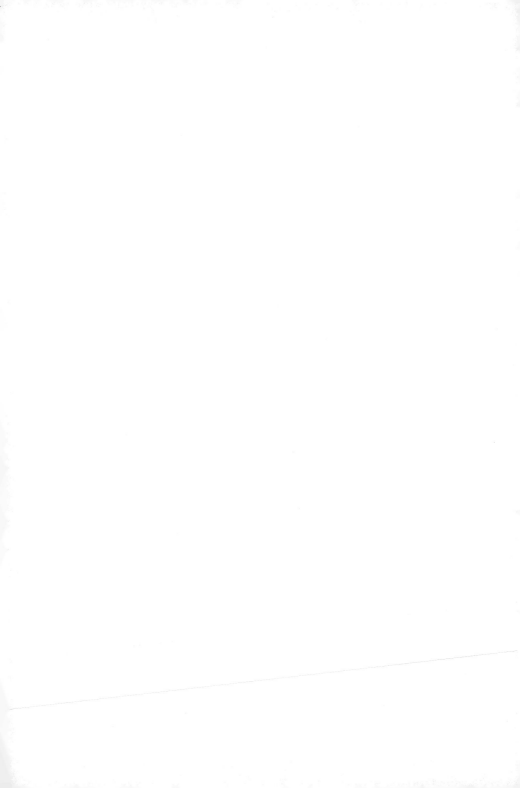

# CONTENTS

# ABBREVIATIONS

AFL-CIO American Federation of Labour–Congress of Industrial
Organizations (1955), union federation.

APHP Assistance Publique–Hôpitaux de Paris (1849) is a set of 38 public
hospitals mostly in Paris but also further.

ARS Agence régionale de santé (2010). A regional health agency (ARS)
is a public administrative establishment of the French State in
charge of the implementation of health policy in its region.

CFDT Confédération Française Démocratique du Travail (1964), French
union confederation, split of the CFTC.

CFTC Confédération Française des Travailleurs Chrétiens (1919), French
and Christian union confederation.

CGT Confédération Générale du Travail (1898), first French union
confederation.

CMU The complementary universal health coverage (1999) is called
'Complémentaire santé solidaire' since 2019. It is a French social
protection scheme that provides access to care and reimbursement
of treatment, benefits and medicines to anyone living in France who
is not already covered by another compulsory health
insurance scheme.

DARES The Direction de l'Animation de la Recherche, des Études et des
Statistiques (Dares) is a department of the French central public
administration, which depends on the Ministry of Labour. It
produces, analyses, studies and statistics on the themes of work,
employment, vocational training and social dialogue.

FO Force Ouvrière (1947), French union federation, split of the CGT.

GDP Gross domestic product is a monetary measure of the market value
of all the final goods and services produced and sold (not resold) in
a specific time period by countries.

| | |
|---|---|
| HAS | Haute autorité en santé (2004), independent scientific public health authority. |
| HPST | Hospital, Patients, Health and Territories Act of 21 July 2009, which transformed the Regional Hospitalisation Agencies (ARH) into Regional Health Agencies (ARS). |
| INSEE | The National Institute of Statistics and Economic Studies is responsible for the production, analysis and publication of official statistics in France since 1946. |
| OECD | The Organisation for Economic Co-operation and Development (1961) is an international organisation for economic studies, whose member countries—mostly developed countries—share a democratic system of government and a market economy. |
| RTT | Réduction du temps de travail (2008), a law that allows employers to pay employees who work more than the legal working time of 35 hours per week with paid holidays. |
| SUD | Solidaires, Unitaires et Démocratiques (1989), union first created in Post and Telecom (SUD-PTT), split of the CFDT, member of the new *Solidaires* federation (1998). |
| T2A or TAA | The Tarification à l'activité (2007) is a method of financing French health establishments resulting from the hospital reform of the 2007 Hospital Plan, which, according to its promoters, aimed to medicalise financing while balancing the allocation of financial resources and giving responsibility to the health players. |
| UNSA | Union Nationale des Syndicats Autonomes (1993), union federation created by five non-confederated unions. |
| WHO | The World Health Organization is a specialised agency of the United Nations for public health established in 1948. |

# INTRODUCTION

This book is a reflection on the work of carers as a form of mobilisation. Who has not been struck by the collective zeal at work in our hospitals? One has the impression of seeing people supporting a cause, as much if not more than employees at work. And not only when they mobilise in an exceptional way, with renewed dedication, as was the case during the recent pandemic. The ethical and collective dimension recalls a form of mobilisation rather than just a job. Especially since, as we will see, carers deploy collective strategies that challenge the hierarchy in order to fulfil their ordinary or extraordinary care missions. In a world as hierarchical as the hospital, the researcher is struck by the bonds of solidarity that can be formed there, like in any social movement worthy of the name. If we add the strength of the identification with the group that is forged in care workers' mobilisations, we can grasp the parallel with a social movement even better.

For all that, carers are not militants. They do not fight the system but rather cooperate to keep it going. Of course, this has to do with the ambivalence of public service missions such as health, which are part of the prerogatives of the state system, but with a different democratic openness. So, while the police and the justice system can be suspected of primarily protecting property owners, and while taxes are primarily based on salaries, the same cannot be said of the hospital, which primarily protects people. Just as the Post Office was admired by the early socialists, who saw it as a public organisation prefiguring a new society, the public hospital and its carers are popular, as the applause heard during the pandemic reminded us. Nurses and firemen regularly top popularity polls, even if the pandemic did not change the social order, neither in France (Sainsaulieu,

2021a) nor in other countries, on the contrary: health workers at the frontline faced a double risk of infection (People's Health Movement, 2021).

However, carers are not naïve. While they cooperate to the best of their ability, they also raise their voices against public underfunding and deteriorating working conditions. They are regularly caught in a dilemma: to cooperate as best they can for the patients or to refuse to cooperate with the system that degrades care for the patients. These are the states of mind we have taken as our object, at least in their collective forms.

In doing so, we accept a certain degree of uncertainty. Taking the collective mobilisation of carers as our object does not only imply grasping its two sides, the consensual and protest aspects. The question of its sociological boundaries is just as important: even though the paramedical care workforce is the most important group in terms of numbers, can we completely leave out doctors, on the one hand, and non-healthcare workers, on the other? Everything depends on the aim, and the aim varies necessarily when we start with an abstract concept that is entirely predefined or with a more flexible conceptual input such as mobilisation. So the target population is variable, depending on whether we are dealing with the professional aspect, where doctors are central and nurses are more specifically concerned than care assistants in the paramedical corps; the trade union aspect, where all hospital workers are involved, and more broadly the middle and working classes; the care aspect, as work where women are in the vast majority, or the care unit or department, where nurses and care assistants most often work together.

Similarly, is the mobilisation of care workers an ordinary or extraordinary phenomenon? Both, of course, because while structural features characterise international hospital work, institutional configurations also weigh heavily, such as the degree of state centralisation and frontal challenges to the state. We will, therefore, endeavour to follow our dependence on the French institutional pathway, where we conducted the majority of our surveys, but in the course of the text, we will make forays into other national contexts, drawing on the available literature. Similarly, while the pandemic will be our focus, we see it more as an indicator of a more general and ordinary phenomenon—healthcare mobilisation.

## METHODOLOGY

This book is based on the results of surveys conducted over a period of 20 years in various types of private and public establishments. Most of the hospitals studied were in France, in different regions of northern, eastern, western and central France. People from all kinds of occupations and professions were interviewed, from ordinary employees to directors and physicians, mostly in qualitative surveys, in a total of more than 600 interviews during 20 years. As previously outlined (Sainsaulieu, 2012, 2021b), our analysis is based on successive surveys on labour relations in hospitals.

The first survey focused on hospitals, on the notion of a local context, by reconstructing social worlds based on an analysis of organised labour relations. The actors themselves are aware of the imprint their 'departments' make on their practice, but they attribute the 'atmosphere' in the latter to a single boss or to the medical specialty and not to collective ways of working (Sainsaulieu, 2006). The second survey, on paramedical participation during accreditation procedures, showed striking examples of staff mobilisation during the development of treatment protocols for accreditation (Sainsaulieu, 2007). An informal dynamic unfolds in a formal setting, leading to a mobilisation that is paradoxically in accord with the institution, even occasioning greater participation than during confrontational mobilisations under trade union control. The third survey expanded our knowledge of the hospital world from a regional perspective and centred on a professional body. This time the issue of participation arose within consensus meetings that developed recommendations for good medical practice: hospital doctors (in this case in the south-west) took part more often when they felt included, that is to say consulted or represented. The fourth survey allowed us to ascertain the strength of communities in certain departments, where patients are unconscious and in a different context (Ontario, Canada). The fifth survey, based on a double questionnaire completed by managers and staff, showed us the highs and lows of participative management, its mythology, but also its performative strength, with the managers presenting the collective healthcare idea to caregivers (Sainsaulieu, 2008b). The representation dimension, therefore, is added to the practical one.

This survey was also an opportunity to update our work on unionism (Sainsaulieu, 1999) by analysing managers' involvement in trade unions. The next two surveys allowed us to tackle the question of the interactions of hospitals with their environments. Hospital departments interact with each other and intervene in health policies beyond their walls, in a system that nevertheless remains essentially 'hospital-centric'. Finally, very recently we added a survey to compare how emergency care staff mobilise to defend working conditions and how all kinds of care staff mobilised during the pandemic (Sainsaulieu, 2021a; Ridel & Sainsaulieu, 2021). These different elements have fed into a reflection on forms of collective mobilisation in hospitals. We also added three surveys on trade unionism outside hospitals, in the postal and banking industries (Sainsaulieu, 1999,

2014). In fact, it is difficult not to compare unionism in different sectors if we want to throw light on unionism in hospitals.

From an analytical point of view, our grid is inspired as much by the sociology of work and industrial relations as by the sociology of professions, organisations and social movements. It seemed to us that the term 'mobilisation' lent itself well to the hospital field because of its collective, dynamic and elastic nature. Always providing, however, that it is related to the world of work and that it takes on a consensual, non-contentious form, even if this is not without subversive effects on the collective itself.

## BIBLIOGRAPHY

People's Health Movement. (2021). *A Political Economy Analysis of the Impact of Covid-19 Pandemic on Health Workers*. Yale Law School.

Ridel, D., & Sainsaulieu, I. (2021). Démobiliser les soignantes? Logiques spatiales, organisationnelles et institutionnelles à l'hôpital. *Espace et société, 183*(2), 51–66.

Sainsaulieu, I. (1999). Sud-PTT: A Political Trade Unionism? *Industrial Relations, 54*(4), 790–814.

Sainsaulieu, I. (2006). *La communauté de soins en question. Le travail hospitalier face aux enjeux de société*. Lamarre.

Sainsaulieu, I. (2007). *L'hôpital et ses acteurs. Appartenances et égalité*. Belin, Perspectives sociologiques.

Sainsaulieu, I. (2008b). Le cadre animateur: figure fragile d'une conciliation légitime. In I. Sainsaulieu (Dir.), *Les cadres hospitaliers. Représentations et pratiques*. Lamarre.

Sainsaulieu, I. (2012). Collective Mobilisation in Hospitals: Confrontational or Consensual? *Revue française de sociologie (English), 53*(3), 316–346.

Sainsaulieu, I. (2014). Retour sur la notion de 'base syndicale'. Le milieu de la CGT des banques en tensions. *L'Homme et la Société*, n°193–194, juin–décembre, 13–41.

Sainsaulieu, I. (2021a). Mobilisations soignantes par gros temps: quelle prise de risque organisationnelle? Point de vue, *Revue française des affaires sociales*, n°4, 97–109.

Sainsaulieu, I. (2021b). Over-mobilisation, Poor Integration of Care Groups: The French Hospital System in the Face of the Pandemic. *Forum for Social Economics, 13*(1), 207–219.

CHAPTER 1

# Structural Limits and Consensual Mobilisation

**Abstract** Despite all the most developed public systems, the health system appears to be under great pressure. All over the world, the work of professionals is constrained by the lack of sufficient staff, the growing needs of an ageing population and the desire to reduce costs by relying on the reduction of the wage bill rather than on the income of independent doctors. The French system is original precisely in that it illustrates the contrast between a centralised state strongly invested in the hospital system and the existence of an equally strong liberal medicine. In a particularly demanding context for healthcare work, we question the meaning of healthcare mobilisation, between adherence to the values of care and the ability to defend them on a daily basis.

**Keywords** Mobilisation • Socialisation • Care • Participatory management • Quality of care

Is there an international dimension to healthcare mobilisation? The question deserves attention. Any academic contribution is necessarily situated geographically but at the same time aspires to universal validity, at the cost of walking an uneasy line: on the one hand, there is a risk of falling into particularism, even though transversal dimensions are attested in the literature. On the other hand, there is the risk of drowning sectoral particularities in an overly broad whole.

On the one hand, it is obvious that mobilisation emerges from a national institutional context, according to different variables, for example, the weight of the public sector, the status of the professions or the role of the hospital within the health system. For this reason, we will be presenting the French context in this introduction, which is the framework for most of our investigations into labour relations in hospitals. Later on, we will also have to specify the context of industrial relations, in particular the role played by trade unions in mobilising healthcare workers.

On the other hand, we could dilute the mechanisms of care work into those of salaried work in general, since in France, as in most countries in the North, most care work is salaried. Care work has become an important part of salaried work, which is now essentially tertiary and is classified, in particular, as a service activity. It is thus related to all activities involving contact with users or customers. It also presents points of comparison with other aspects of salaried work, via the productivist pressure increasingly characterising working conditions in the hospital world, which carers have been telling us for years resembles work on a production line ('it's a real factory!'). Finally, like standardised airport work, hospital work has internationally shared structural features, due to the necessarily specialised medical organisation, to a standardised stratification between carers and non-carers, between doctors and paramedics, between administrative and medical hierarchies, not to mention hygiene and safety standards.

For all these reasons, it is difficult to distinguish the local from the general. Invariably, even the most quantitative comparative analyses are accused of leaving out whole sections of the reality of the North or the South, the West or the East. This is not our methodology, which is essentially qualitative, possibly inspired by monographs carried out in Canada (Ontario) or Switzerland, or quantitative, but focused on France (*see methodology above*). So, we will endeavour to provide contextualising elements on a case-by-case basis, drawing on the literature on care work and hospital organisation, trade unionism and social movements. It is essential for the reader, who has experience and expertise, to interpret the text in such a way as to be able to judge its scope.

## 1.1    INDIVIDUAL VOCATIONS AND SOCIALISATION IN CARE WORK

In France, the commitment of carers during the first wave of the pandemic was much praised. Supporting those who are fighting disease and death seems to make sense, and nurses and firefighters do not need special events to be popular.

Yet, there are two ways to understand this popularity. The first is moral. Those who show compassion deserve compassion. Seemingly Christian, this morality exists in other traditions as well, and the legitimacy of care continues when religion disappears from the hospital and society. Instead of religion invading morality, it is morality that invades religion, and it is morality that maintains itself after religion has withdrawn. We now speak of ethical issues, or even ethical committees, attached to hospital structures. Ethics and morality are not necessarily distinct concepts, but ethics committees try to shed light on delicate cases, by trying to stand back and consider all parameters. These cases may also extend into the legal sphere—hence the interest for the institution of examining the problems ahead of time in order to prevent them. In philosophical terms, Cynthia Fleury sees care as a humanism, particularly sensitive to the vulnerability of others. Like others, she advocates a more egalitarian relationship between doctor and patient, and a refocusing of caregivers on the purpose of their action. However, care is not just a moral issue: it even has a particularly developed social component.

Indeed, hospitals are also increasingly an economic issue, in terms of jobs, salaries, markets, private profits and public taxes. Sometimes health is expensive, and sometimes it is 'priceless', as Macron said during the pandemic. It is set free from economic issues only to fall back into them and vice versa. Sometimes it is a professional matter, whose ethics escape the economy (as in the Hippocratic oath, the paragon of medical disinterestedness); sometimes it is a budgetary matter, in which every medical expense must be controlled by the public administration; sometimes it is a business, where the state must pay a high price for drugs to private laboratories. We will return to this later.

Money is also present among the concerns of doctors, as we shall see. What is certain is that the work cannot enrich the mass of other workers, paramedics or ordinary hospital staff. It is true that for young people worried about their professional future job security plays a role in their choice to work in a state hospital. But the increase in vocations following the pandemic shows that job security is not the only concern, on the contrary: the health risk incurred should have dissuaded new vocations in this case.

So who are these carers who are dedicated to patients? From their point of view, female carers are not saints who sacrifice themselves for the patient. In this respect, they readily differentiate themselves from the 'old-timers', nuns and the like, who 'would have thrown themselves out of the window' if the doctor had asked them to.

The mediation of the doctor is significant: it indicates an organisation of work, a hierarchy and a division of tasks, in contradiction with the pure register of the vocation or motivation to care.

Work is indeed at the heart of care. The motivation for choosing to be a carer is certainly prior to employment, but the theme of personal vocation tends to refer all motivation to family upbringing. Here again, we must be careful.

Firstly, it is less as individuals than as a gender that women are assigned to care work. There are certainly particular subsets, such as those caring families where several members sometimes work in the same establishment. But the vast majority of nurses and care assistants are women. Although women have made inroads into all sorts of professions and careers that were once alien to them, they are still overwhelmingly assigned to the caring professions, in other words, to taking care of others, looking after the elderly or supervising and educating children, in hospitals or schools, in healthcare or social work.

Individual motivation also changes. By becoming professional, a female employee becomes more independent. She gains more financial independence, from her family or in her relationship. And by working, she more or less transforms her vision of the world. Professional socialisation can change behaviour, occupations, concerns and relationships. Many couples are formed at work, through professional endogamy. In the course of one's career, the content of professional interest changes. While young people are passionate about or absorbed by training, technical gestures and tools, and the unit or department to which they are assigned, older people take a step back and look more closely at the context: work relations, work organisation, changes in the hospital and public health. Moreover, the recurrent problems of the hospital affect them all: men and women, young and old, are all concerned about the lack of staff and the promises of the health minister. Working in a hospital is politicised in the sense that individuals take part in a vast and organised social body, which broadens their horizons and reveals antagonisms within a state entity that their professional orientation in the national health service, like their inclination to care for others, willingly led them to believe was entirely at the service of patients.

Changes in outlook do not always reflect a maturing judgement of the hospital experience. Many people change direction during their professional careers: they specialise or become supervisors, retire from work for family reasons, find another job as a nurse in a different administration, or even in an associative or private framework, not to mention those who change medical departments or public establishments. In all, a nurse's career lasts less than ten years.

However, this internal or external mobility does not prevent two-thirds of nurses from being grouped together in hospitals, where they account for the largest category of staff in general and of care workers in particular, including doctors. This is why it is not absurd to ask how they forge a collective identity and consciousness and how this relates to the fate of society as a whole. Are nurses and care assistants the new working-class heroes? We will see why they have every reason to be, without reducing the complexity of their experiences.

## 1.2   THE FRENCH HEALTH SYSTEM: CENTRAL GOVERNMENT AND PRIVATE HEALTHCARE

Like other systems, the French health service has taken a managerial turn, under pressure from social and economic forces (Sainsaulieu, 2021b). Reputed to be exemplary, following the measures taken to create a welfare state in 1945, the French system has been reformed several times, not without consequences for the working conditions of carers. At the turn of the century, all international studies (EU, OECD, WHO) affirmed that France had one of the best-performing health systems in the world. Accessible to the entire population via compulsory health insurance, this system combines the latter with complementary schemes and solidarity mechanisms such as universal health coverage (CMU) or assistance in acquiring complementary healthcare (ACS). In principle, the French system is one of the most generous in terms of coverage, at the cost of a significant weight in GDP: 12% in 2012, and 11.3% in 2018. The average for OECD countries was 8.8% in 2017.

In Germany, spending is the same in percentage terms, but as GDP is higher, public spending per capita is also higher, with, for example, twice as many acute care beds: six per thousand instead of three per thousand in France. The percentage expenditure on hospitals and hospital administration is higher in France, whereas the expenditure on ambulatory medicine, drugs and prevention is higher in Germany.

The French model is indeed characterised by the traditional confrontation between the central state and private healthcare, in contrast to the decentralised self-administration of German health funds and the traditional association of the German medical profession with the management of the health system. Recent developments confirm the institutional trajectory in France: although doctors joined the hospital as it became more powerful after the Debré reform in 1959, they have always retained the option of private activity and have tended to take refuge in private clinics in the face of increasing problems in the public hospital. On the other hand, the rise of social and health taxation (Generalised Social Contribution, Universal Health Coverage), the influence of Parliament (which votes each year on financing Social Security) and the administrative influence on hospital medical activity have only increased the role of the state.

The French impulse to reform reactivates these structural contradictions. For the national health conference of 18 June 2013, the organisation of care needed to be simplified, decompartmentalised and refocused around patients and their GPs in a territory and along pathways where individuals are given more responsibility. Financing universal health protection is also based on residential criteria, as well as on organising care through doctors outside the hospital, in order to prevent unnecessary hospitalisations. The regionalisation of healthcare has been one of the major thrusts of hospital and health policies, through the implementation of the Hospital, Patients, Health and Territories (HPST) Act of 21 July 2009, which transformed the Regional Hospitalisation Agencies (ARH) into Regional Health Agencies (ARS) from 1 April 2010. In practice, these new structures assert administrative power at the regional level, whereas the T2A reform in 2004 had reaffirmed administrative power at the national level.

*A Health Business Integrating the State and the Market*
The record of the reforms has been severely criticised for, among other things, concentrating power in the hands of the administration to the benefit of private social forces. In a collective article (Leicht et al., 2009), we noted that the French health system seems to follow the trend of

subjecting the medical professions to new governance structures inspired by the free market. The new public management represents a hybrid between the pluralist concerns of the state and a context where the role of the state is challenged by the multiplication of players, especially private players. Through the health agencies created from the 1990s onwards, the state's domination of healthcare had to deal with this pluralism in order to focus on the provision of health services.

Market pressures are considerable. Colleagues have pointed out that healthcare is a huge financial windfall that many companies would like to capture. In 2017, the 'consumption of care and medical goods' (CSBM) amounted to 199.3 billion euros, 77.8% of which was financed by compulsory health insurance (Social Security). The CSBM is made up of expenditure on hospital care (46.6%) and outpatient care (53.4%), which includes, in particular, medical and dental consultations, as well as expenditure on drugs (Abecassis et al., 2019, pp. 142–150). According to the ONDAM (the official health expenditure indicator), the share of hospital care spending has indeed fallen as a result of policies aimed at saving money, but not the share of outpatient care: it has even decreased in favour of 'outpatient care', while care outside hospitals is failing to fulfil its missions of accessibility, in particular by refusing disadvantaged patients, even though they are covered by the CMU (Askenazy et al., 2013). Clearly, the control of health expenditure weighs more heavily on the hospital sector than on private practice.

The state and the market are growing in parallel: while a new management bureaucracy is developing in the health system like elsewhere (Hibou, 2012), pharmaceutical firms and complementary health insurers are the big winners in the weakening of social security and the de-socialisation of a growing amount of health spending. The exorbitant prices of drugs are jeopardising the reimbursement systems for the benefit of company shareholders. The market logic in the health system results in rationing treatments for certain pathologies, deteriorating care and working conditions in hospitals (Sainsaulieu, 2003) and higher contributions from patients (Askenazy et al., 2013). This is the case in the US, where spending amounts to 16% of GDP, without guaranteeing better access to healthcare, and increasingly in France, where the delisting of certain drugs or care (such as dental care, which is poorly covered) discourages access to treatment and increases health inequalities (Dubost, Pollack, & Rey, 2020). A shortage of doctors has increased the cost of ex-hospital doctors, who have become freelancers working at high rates per half day in public hospitals.

## The Reform Steamroller

At the professional level, new management and financing methods have gradually stifled a hospital-centred system decried for its cost and complexity. One would have thought that medical authority, with its parliamentary political affinities, would have been able to resist the management wave. Traditionally important, medical authority has weakened. For a time, the hospital-academic elite waged 'open war' but had to give in, showing 'the vulnerability of the professional worlds to the process of managerial integration'. Indeed, some have taken advantage of the reform to rise in the hierarchy, while others have chosen the private medicine route to benefit from the industrialisation of hospital medicine in their medical speciality. Big bosses as much as healthcare workers had to give in to the administrative elite of finance inspectors 'flanked by consultants' from prestigious (and expensive) consultancies. Hospital reform has thus taken a distinctly top-down turn that contradicts the idea of pluralism embodied by models of governance with a democratic tone.

Similarly, the other hospital players did not form a united opposition against the reforms because the new public management divided them according to their capacity to adapt, creating opportunities for some and not for others. Above all, they have suffered the full force of measures to reduce the wage bill, generating savings in the health accounts at the expense of the public hospital in general and the work of carers in particular: from the 1990s onwards, measures such as reducing the length of hospital stays were introduced, the direct result of which was an increase in the work rate for carers due to the increased turnover of patients in beds without compensatory recruitment (Sainsaulieu, 2003, 2007). In Switzerland, the average length of stay in acute care services was reduced by about two days in 20 years (2002–2019), from seven to five days. In France, in 2014, despite the progress made, the healthcare insurance fund was still recommending making 'savings of 3 billion euros over 3 years'.

Empirical analyses conducted from the mid-2000s onwards, mainly based on qualitative field surveys, show an 'increasing pressure on work rate' between 1998 and 2013, with a clear acceleration between 2005 and

2013 (Gheorghiu & Moatty, 2013, p. 250). This pressure is accompanied by a deterioration in working conditions in the hospital sector (Sainsaulieu, 2003). However, these trends are not specific to the hospital sector but can be observed for all sectors over the same period: colleagues thus highlight a resumption of work intensification for all workers between 2005 and 2013, after a stabilisation between 1998 and 2005, to which is added an increase in physical constraints and tensions at work.

Nevertheless, this increase in physical constraints is significantly greater for workers in the hospital sector, who are now very heavily exposed to rising work rates linked to compliance with production standards or deadlines, or to dependence on the work of one or more colleagues. The implementation of the reduction in working hours (RTT) has, as in other sectors, generated perverse effects leading to a deterioration in working conditions. The reduction or even absence of recruitment has encouraged a process of work intensification. In other words, while the number of hours worked has decreased, the work has intensified. On this point, the hospital has evolved like other productive sectors: the reduction in working hours has resulted in intensified, more flexible and versatile work. The introduction of the T2A has also reinforced the intensification of work.

Over the period from 2003 to 2009, the increase in activity in public healthcare establishments was faster than the increase in healthcare personnel. Hospital productivity increased by 11.3% over this period, or 1.8% a year. The increase was even more marked between 2007 and 2008, the year of the transition to T2A as the sole means of financing hospitals. The absolute quest for productivity is reflected in a growing reduction in staff numbers, pressure on carers and increasing flexibility. This logic accentuates all kinds of constraints on staff: changes in working hours, time overruns, difficulties in the free choice of holidays, tougher management of the health system or recalling nurses on leave to work (Gheorghiu & Moatty, 2013). Although the increased time pressure of hospital work is accompanied by a slight easing of the 'historical' constraints of the hospital, particularly physical and time constraints, in 2013 workers in this sector were even more often subject to at least one form of staggered working hours, physical hardship and constraints in the work environment (Benallah & Domin, 2017). This has led to a deterioration in occupational health, with an increase in stress and back illnesses (Benallah & Domin, 2017).

The situation in the US is comparable in terms of deteriorating working conditions. Looking at the causes of burnout, a recent literature review identified the most common ones: '*we first identified high workload, value incongruence, low control over work, low decision latitude, poor social climate/support, and low rewards as predictors of burnout*' (Dall'Ora et al., 2020). These factors were consistent with the authors' working hypothesis. They later added others: '*Other factors have been classified as predictors of burnout in the nursing literature: 'low/inappropriate nurse staffing levels, 12-hour workdays, low schedule flexibility, time pressure, high job and psychological demands, low task variety, role conflict, low autonomy, negative nurse-physician relationship, poor supervisor/leader support, poor leadership, negative team relationship and job insecurity*' (Dall'Ora et al., 2020). While the range seems somewhat broad and imprecise, it gives a good qualitative idea of the observable disruptions in daily work practices.

## 1.3    PARTICIPATORY MANAGEMENT AROUND QUALITY OF CARE

In the past, the top-down approach to reform had to give way to the specificities of professional work and common sense. It had to revert to participatory mechanisms, either to counter big bosses' power to harm in the workplace or to motivate staff and respond to the many contradictions between individual quality of patient care and managerial standards (Sainsaulieu, 2007).

As a professional bureaucracy, the social world of the hospital has always been constructed through a negotiated social order, particularly, in France, between administrative and medical powers, rather than with patients (Mintzberg, 1982; Strauss, 1992; R. Sainsaulieu, 1999). The desire for reform has clearly shown a shift in emphasis from the public service to the market, both as an external entity and as an internal operating mode. However, in no modern organisation are so many professionals concentrated in the same workplaces.

Improving the quality of care has been a leitmotif for maintaining a virtuous confusion between budgetary rationality, over-emphasis on the private sector and professional foundations: does not quality imply both the economy of means in relation to the goal sought and the respect for professional standards? Cooperation between professionals has been encouraged within the framework of 'city-hospital coordination' and 'health democracy'. Support for the creation of multi-professional teams, organised around the attending physician and in conjunction with the hospital and specialised care, has been made a priority. The law (HPST) has thus provided several incentives for cooperation, networking of health players and the emergence of real comprehensive care for patients. As a result, numerous mobile teams have been set up outside or within hospitals, for example, in the field of palliative care and geriatrics (Castra & Sainsaulieu, 2020).

Within the hospital, our investigations showed that nurses experienced collective accountability, that nursing managers were created as guarantors of quality assurance, and that doctors had to cooperate with management arrangements.

As far as nurses are concerned, a collective approach has prevailed, particularly in the context of hospital accreditation, a participatory process which they appreciate and which in turn makes them feel valued (Sainsaulieu, 2012). The participants mentioned a broadening of their horizons, the development of professional and organisational awareness, the habit of self-assessment and targeted accountability (assigning responsibility for a particular aspect of work to specific employees).

The first condition for success was the existence of close links between the evaluative logic of accreditation and the professional and organisational logic of nurses. The nurses were (more or less) responsible for coordinating care in their unit and were sometimes in conflict with the doctors over the control of patients. The second precondition was the existence of links between health professionals before the accreditation process. Smaller units with strong, dynamic collectives and good performance measures were better able to make collective assessments of accreditation. Success was limited by the lack of time available for collective decision-making and the decline in enthusiasm over time due to fatigue.

Middle managers were very supportive of the quality assessment process (Sainsaulieu, 2008). More specifically, middle managers saw themselves as serving patients and professionals in the name of healthcare quality, the overarching objective of the French hospital accreditation system. To what extent does financial management mean quality management? Managers were in favour of the new accreditation guidelines because they saw themselves as guarantors of quality healthcare, even if they had to focus on the financial aspect. Middle managers tend to be appreciated by the staff. While the quality of management varies in the eyes of the nursing staff, it is not uncommon to hear nurses praising the 'good' managers in the department. In an earlier survey, 51% of the nurses interviewed considered their immediate supervisors to be 'useful', especially in arbitrating their differences, although they rejected their claim to be 'part of the team' (Sainsaulieu, 2008).

Most of the time, managers and doctors on the ward felt close to the difficulties faced by the nursing staff. Doctors have also been included in the new evaluation procedures. While medical quality assurance in France was based on moral and professional control and continuing education (a legal obligation since 1996), under the supervision of the *Haute Autorité en Santé* (HAS), more good practice guidelines were developed by consensus conferences (a meeting of experts to reach a common decision on a medical problem). The evaluation involved collecting information, choosing a reference group, self-assessment, writing the individual assessment and sending it to the authorities, a summary meeting in which the doctor proposes ideas for his or her own improvement, and a confidential report written and sent to the doctor with proposals for further training. However, through the normative control of the HAS (Haute Autorité en Santé), the state has mainly relied on professional standards to keep doctors in line with new regulations.

Nonetheless, participatory management has two limits, temporal and formal. It is more or less strong depending on the period, giving way to top-down management processes in the later period. Furthermore, it does not in itself summarise the range in which collective care energy is deployed, in other words the forms of care mobilisation.

## 1.4   What Kind of Healthcare Mobilisation?

How have healthcare workers reacted collectively to the new work constraints? In the French context, the question of healthcare workers and the trade unions must be dealt with separately. The particularity of the mobilisation of healthcare workers is that it has a form of autonomy in relation to the hierarchical and trade union framework. Without being the work of a profession, or even a semi-profession of nursing, nursing mobilisation is composite. It is based on cooperation between various professions at different levels of the social scale, and is sometimes more moderate, sometimes more radical than traditional trade union mobilisation. It expresses the multiple facets of the collective work of carers, its working-class and middle-class social components, its admiration for doctors or its wage anchoring, its multiple forms of identification with other workers (from the nurse-assistant pair to the medical department, or even the entire hospital establishment), and its different age strata. It does not form a homogeneous whole and, depending on the moment, its boundaries widen or narrow, sometimes including doctors, for example, and sometimes hospital staff. Its political significance is no clearer, because it sometimes reproduces the traditional role of care, while sometimes it sets up this care as a new social model, providing the world with an ethical response to its afflictions; sometimes it appears as enlightened work, with an avant-garde civilising mission, and sometimes it shows work in its most oppressive light, that of assembly-line work.

This is why it does not fit into the established grid of sociological models. It is neither professional in the strict sense (nurses have never managed to form a separate profession in France), nor classist in the pure sense, nor is it the expression of a field, in the Bourdieusian sense of the term. While medicine can be interpreted as a field, historically constructed by doctors (Pinell, 2009), the same cannot be said for this dynamic body of carers with changing contours. Nor is it a question of a linked ecology, the parallel construction of an internal profession with an external ally (Abbott, 1988). Nor is it a social movement, because the mobilisation of care workers usually takes place inside the hospital and does not necessarily involve a protest claim. On the other hand, it is not a routine mobilisation either, comparable to ordinary work. In the definition we have given of it, healthcare mobilisation brings about a local transformation of social relations in a more egalitarian direction (Sainsaulieu, 2012). Like all collective work, it gives impetus to a dynamic in which everyone has a place, from the stretcher-bearer to the head doctor, and where even the head doctor speaks on behalf of everyone. However, it does not always follow the limits of the healthcare service: competing medical logics and their symbolic divisions only partially rub off on healthcare work, just as even lower-level hospital managers are only partially members of the healthcare work team in the eyes of its membership. Can we then speak of a single phenomenon and a coherent social fact, or is care mobilisation merely an aggregate of disparate elements? This is what we will examine in the following chapters.

In order to consider its specific nature, we felt it was important to compare it to trade unions in the hospital. The trade union traditionally embodies a collective group. But in France at least, this group is strongly dissociated from the union, and this is not specific to the hospital world, but it is even truer in the world of healthcare. Paradoxically, while the aim of trade unionism is to bring together various professions, the world of healthcare seems richer. The second chapter emphasises the territorial roots of this caring world, which can drastically limit its scope, since it assigns it to a given place. This particular place can only be relativised by the trade unionist, who refers more generally to the world of work. However, service is at the heart of healthcare mobilisation, even if it sometimes limits individual horizons. In the third chapter trade unionism will appear to be particularly disembodied, driven by the institution rather than by concrete social groups. We will see in particular how the notion of the union base is ambivalent, referring sometimes to the union's affiliates and sometimes to the reference company environment, with a gap between the two. The fourth chapter will be an opportunity to analyse the different forms of alternative models of healthcare with different meanings of care, the service society, and some more practical experiments. Finally, we will examine the comparative roles of self-organised healthcare autonomy and trade unionism in concrete protest mobilisations, particularly on the occasion of the 2019 emergency room strike.

## BIBLIOGRAPHY

Abbott, A. (1988). *The System of Professions*. University of Chicago Press.

Abecassis, P., Coutinet, N., Juven, P., & Vincent, F. (2019). La santé, un business? In: Fondation Copernic (Éd.), *Manuel indocile de sciences sociales: Pour des savoirs résistants* (pp. 142–150). La Découverte.

Askenazy, P., Dormont, B., Geoffard, P., & Paris, V. (2013). Pour un système de santé plus efficace. *Notes du conseil d'analyse économique, 8*, 1–12.

Benallah, S., & Domin, J.-P. (2017). Intensité et pénibilités du travail à l'hôpital. *Travail et Emploi* [En ligne], 152 | octobre–décembre, mis en ligne le 01 octobre 2019. http://journals.openedition.org/travailemploi/7755

Castra, M., & Sainsaulieu, I. (2020). Intervenir sur un autre territoire professionnel. Equipes mobiles et services sédentaires à l'hôpital. *Sciences sociales et santé, 38*(4), 47–74.

Dall'Ora, C., Ball, J., Reinius, M., & Griffiths, P. (2020, June 5). Burnout in Nursing: A Theoretical Review. *Human Resource Health, 18*(1), 41.

Dubost, Cl., Pollack, C., & Rey, S. (2020). Les inégalités sociales face à l'épidémie de Covid-19. *Les dossiers de la DREE*, n° 62.

Gheorghiu, M. D., & Moatty, F. (2013). L'hôpital en mouvement. Changements organisationnels et conditions de travail: Rueil-Malmaison, éditions Liaisons, [Noisy-le-Grand], Centre d'études de l'emploi, coll. "Liaisons sociales".

Hibou, B. (2012). *La bureaucratisation du monde à l'ère néolibérale*. La Découverte.

Leicht, K. T., Walter, T., Sainsaulieu, I., & Davies, S. (2009). New Public Management and New Professionalism across Nations and Contexts. In New Governance and New Professionalism, n° spécial, *Current Sociology*, Sage, *57*(4), 581–605.

Mintzberg, H. (1982). *Structures et dynamiques d'organisation.* Editions d'organisation.

Pinell, P. (2009). La genèse du champ médical: le cas de la France (1795–1870). *Revue française de sociologie, 50*(2), 315–349.

Sainsaulieu, I. (1999). Sud-PTT: A Political Trade Unionism? *Industrial Relations, 54*(4), 790–814.

Sainsaulieu, I. (2003). *Le malaise des soignants. Le travail sous pression à l'hôpital.* L'Harmattan.

Sainsaulieu, I. (2007). *L'hôpital et ses acteurs. Appartenances et égalité.* Belin, Perspectives sociologiques.

Sainsaulieu, I. (2008). Le syndicalisme à l'hôpital. Sociologie d'une insatisfaction. Dossier Syndicalisme et santé, *Les Tribunes de la santé*, n°18, 83–94.

Sainsaulieu, I. (2012). Collective Mobilisation in Hospitals: Confrontational or Consensual? *Revue française de sociologie (English), 53*(3), 316–346.

Sainsaulieu, I. (2020). Les Gilets jaunes, un peuple sans classes? Lectures critiques. *Revue française de science politique, 70*, 271–286.

Sainsaulieu, I. (2021b). Over-mobilisation, Poor Integration of Care Groups: The French Hospital System in the Face of the Pandemic. *Forum for Social Economics, 13*(1), 207–219.

CHAPTER 2

# The Roots of Healthcare

**Abstract** In the hospital, it is by analysing the cultures of the care service that we can understand the professional socialisation of carers. There are territories that obey traditions born of the necessities of cooperation at work. Thus, some particular working conditions, where interdependence between colleagues is required at the heart of daily practices, create a collective more than in other care units. They are generally referred to as closed departments, emphasising their hygienic isolation, whereas the sociological survey rather emphasises the modalities of closer cooperation. The doctors are caught up in the strongest cultures but they identify more with a cross-sectional medical professional body. These care service cultures have advantages and disadvantages, which we examine in more detail here.

**Keywords** Territorial roots • Pandemic • Doctors identities • Healthcare closures

Individual vocation is often the explanation put forward by carers for their commitment. In the media in particular, they justify sacrificing leave or the health risks involved: '*if you have chosen this profession, it is not for nothing*'. The implication is that you have to accept the risks, and these risks have been accepted for a long time. Is the nursing profession the result of a 'vocation', that is, a straight trajectory marked by a kind of predestination? Let us consider this point.

Of course, some people may have dreamed of becoming nurses from childhood. But it is not just an individual vocation, as we saw before. Collectively, women are predestined by their primary education to the care professions, where they are in a majority. On the other hand, this sacrificial discourse, which can arise more strongly at certain times, is not part of the daily life of women carers. In France, no one goes to work singing about saving humankind or their homeland. In previous writings, I have referred to the recurring issue of public service, to underline the intermittent scope of the sense of mission (Sainsaulieu, 2007). It is certain that the carers who volunteered to go to the 'covidated' services must have felt their mission was important. However, this feeling is unevenly shared, either diachronically (otherwise commitment would not be stronger in times of pandemic) or synchronically, as not everyone volunteers. Not all carers are touched by grace, even if they are often admirable.

One way out of the 'mystery of grace', an old theological debate, is to look more closely at professional socialisation. What is happening at work that can give professional meaning to carers? In the introduction, we saw how the relationship of the carer to technique and to organisational changes in the course of her individual career, that is, as a function of her career progression. Here we would like to focus on the collective sense of work, which has certainly matured over time, but which is identical for all carers, even if it is not felt to the same degree according to this advancement and according to the type of department to which they are attached.

A good way of understanding this is to look at the collective dimension in nursing discourse, in other words, the uses of 'we'. Whom do they mean when they say we? It is on this point that we will dwell, taking the case of nurses and doctors in turn. The 'department' (administratively, it has become the care unit, but those involved continue to refer to 'their department') is undoubtedly the first point of attachment for the nurses collectively, whereas the medical profession is defined more in terms of a medical professional horizon.

## 2.1   THE TERRITORIAL ROOTS OF HEALTHCARE

The concrete reason why care workers not only have a vocation 'before' employment, but also have a professional sense 'after' employment, is because they are anchored in a 'territory' that shapes them. It is in this context that they can put their learning into practice and translate it into concrete actions that depend not only on the medical or even paramedical speciality but also on the habits of the department. One HR director once told us: '*to change the company culture, you have to wait until the last representative has left*'. In other words, the old-timers can make life difficult for managers. They rule over the department, sometimes constituting such a counter-power that the manager cannot overcome it. Above all, they train the newcomers on the job in the ways they are used to performing their role. Of course, newcomers can eventually make their mark, even building new, broader, more inclusive solidarities or establishing a different working atmosphere, for better or worse. But they will have to wait a while first.

That said, this anchoring is not only customary; it is human. It strongly limits the horizons of carers, so strong is their sense of belonging. So, going to help out colleagues is understood first and foremost at the level of the department, or even within the team that shares the same schedules. The night shift is particularly dependent on solidarity. Indeed, staff are scarce and supervision disappears, leaving the carers isolated in case of a problem. So they need to be able to rely on the nurse working on the floor above or below to come and help out in the event of a problem, if an agitated patient has to be calmed down or even restrained. In the same way, solidarity is more easily expressed when there is a lack of equipment or staff within the same department. It is as if humanity, like all animal species, takes more care of what is close to hand, both in the family and at work. At work, we define a familiar territory within which we have our ties, our concerns, our activity and comfort zone, and above all, our relationships: by seeing the same people, we create reciprocal links, we fraternise, and we humanise our immediate environment more. This frees us from wondering every day whom to have lunch with and above all from the risk of going to eat alone, assuming of course that we have time to eat. This leads to a tendency to think first of the people one knows, and even to cultivate a somewhat chilly, exclusionary peer group. Without necessarily being exclusive, this propensity can sometimes become so, as managers, activists, newcomers or old-timers concerned about the proper functioning of a larger group may regularly regret.

In their quest to establish greater transversality in the way departments work, hospital managers may particularly deplore excessive territoriality. For example, a new system may be introduced to give greater priority to emergency patients. After all, the medical logic of the department is to take patients with specific pathologies and not the general public. Whereas any kind of patient will arrive at the emergency department… More spe-cifically, as regards the patients who arrive in an emergency and need to be hospitalised, many are poly-pathological and suffer from a general deterio-ration linked to delays in medical care, in particular among the elderly, isolated or low-income people. This sometimes general deterioration is not the responsibility of any particular service or of all of them in general, but it serves to widen the gap between the two aspects of medicine, known as both 'general' and 'specialised' medicine, represented in particular in hospitals by the emergency services on the one hand and the specialised care units on the other.

While an excessive sense of belonging is always regrettable, we should not confuse a territory with a burrow! In a professional territory, the matrix is plural and connected. In other words, it is to the extent that the work is done collectively that the feeling of belonging is strong. It is not enough to have walls delimiting a space. Some departments are more appealing than others. Such differences are usually interpreted according to the seriousness of the pathologies, which are supposed to attract more attention from the carers. It is true that patient deaths are unevenly dis-tributed in the hospital and are more common in intensive care units (ICU). Both the ICU and the operating theatre are in fact among the departments where we have seen the most shared identity.

### The Good Patient Is Under Control (Sainsaulieu, 2009)

However, it is not exactly the patient who gives the department its identity but rather its control. The patient tends to differentiate the identities between carers: more often than cleaners or nurses, care assistants mention the relationship with the patient as an important part of their identity. They differentiate themselves by emphasising the comfort of patients, which is their responsibility, as opposed to the 'nurses who give them jabs'. For the cleaning ladies, the pleasure of the patient who is happy to see that the room is clean and 'smells good' is also constitutive but more indirectly: they expect the patient to acknowledge their work.

But the patient does not play the same role at the level of the depart-ment. In our surveys, we saw major contrasts in job satisfaction between departments, which was not due to the relationship with the patient but rather to control. Like a pianist, every professional seeks to master their art. Unlike the pianist, the carer is not dealing with an object (which is already not always easy to master!) but with a patient. Of course, carers work for the patient but 'for' does not mean 'with', even in the cases mentioned above. We know how much doctors have had to change their culture in order to accept dialogue with the patient, and how much they still lack the time or even the desire to do so. For the healthcare team, talking to the patient is even less essential—and they have even less time for it. So the ideal work is done with unconscious patients rather than conscious ones: the good patient is under control. This formula was even used as the title of one of our sociology articles (Sainsaulieu, 2009). Just as the teacher prefers well-behaved pupils, the carer tends to prefer calm patients, and they are never so calm as when they are fully dependent, and therefore unconscious. It is true that carers are moved and challenged by suffering or amusing patients who remind them of their relatives, parents or children. But this interpretation is trying, because it is uncertain: death is lurking. Professionally, you have to know how to manage your emotions, keep the right distance—neither too distant nor too close. Managing one's emotions does not mean trying to stimulate them. You need challenges to test your professional capacity, just as it is better to play tennis with someone better than you. But the challenge is not to be defeated but to win, by showing oneself capable of overcoming adversity. In intensive care, the tension is constant but so is the control.

But this control is collective. Individuals complement each other; they rely on each other. The team bond does not have the same intensity in all departments. But it is in the departments where collaboration is most necessary, where the patient's dependence is strongest, that the feeling of belonging is most marked. This is the equation that we have seen repeatedly in the field. In many departments, collaboration is more limited, and the collective sense of belonging is reduced accordingly. Some identify only with their work partner, a nurse and a care assistant, for example, with whom they constantly work. Others identify with the nurses on the ward, with the doctors, with the patients, with the team (day or night) or with the department as a whole. It all depends on whom the active collaboration is with, and it is more or less inclusive depending on the type of cooperation in the work.

## 2.2    STRENGTHS AND WEAKNESSES OF A DEPARTMENT
## APPROACH IN TIMES OF PANDEMIC[1]

One might think that female carers, devoted to care and always working in a department and in a team, live in a collective work atmosphere, like the medical students in the television series *Hippocrates*, who are particularly festive, joyful, united and even unbridled when they get together. In reality, care workers more often work in pairs (a nurse and a care assistant) and do not always feel solidarity with the entire team. Staff are lucky when this happens.

In intensive care pneumology, A, a young nurse (two years on the ward), clearly feels that she lives in a different group from the others: '*Before I was in the pool of locum nurses, I saw the difference, it's not the same atmosphere in the other pneumology department, which focuses on palliative care. In cardiology, the same, I didn't feel particularly... In cardiac thoracic surgery, there wasn't a very good atmosphere either. You hear gossip...*' (A). As a result, COVID did not change the way the team functioned:

*Between carers I don't really know [whether* COVID *changed things]... we were already a very close team, we have remained the same team without any additional carers, we get on very well, so we help each other if there is a problem, as soon as one of us is more available she asks who needs help. We have always worked like that.* (A)

The collective dynamic exists in some care services that are more cohesive than others. In palliative care, a collective substratum most probably also exists, based on a great deal of listening. '*We are already a fairly autonomous team. We are not in the business of carrying out orders, we are in the business of interacting with the doctors and managers (...). There are always some loudmouths, but people who don't talk much are listened to, we have a very different way of working. We don't do the same job in palliative care. As a result, what people say is always taken into account*', says a palliative care nurse (SP). This reality is unknown to the outside world because

[1] Acknowledgements: this passage (pp. 16–18) is derived from two articles published: Sainsaulieu, I., 2021, 'Mobilisations soignantes par gros temps: quelle prise de risque organisationnelle?', Point de vue, *Revue française des affaires sociales*, n°4, pp. 97–109; Sainsaulieu, I., 2021, *Forum for Social Economics*, 1–13, ©Routledge, Taylor and Francis group, Volume 51 Issue 2, available online: Over-Mobilization, Poor Integration of Care Groups: The French Hospital System in the Face of the Pandemic, via tandfonline.com.

it is counter-intuitive: '*People have the impression that it is a very sad department, when in fact it is not, it is one of the liveliest departments I have ever worked in*'.

On the other hand, this experienced woman, who is also a trade unionist, does not idealise her department. She finds limits to the mutual empathy. '*In our department, there is solidarity within the team but not with colleagues from other departments in our unit. The team does not deny that others have difficulties, but we do not push our solidarity to the point of seeing if the neuro needs us. We know that geriatrics has deplorable working conditions but that's all. For example, a few years ago, geriatric colleagues went on strike because of working conditions, and I proposed to make a gesture, but I was not listened to*' (SP).

And what about the ability of new staff to integrate into the department team? Moving to another department is often a challenge. In the case of intra-hospital mobile teams, which travel to visit patients in other departments, the 'nomads' are often perceived as intrusive by the 'sedentary' staff of the department visited (Castra & Sainsaulieu, 2020). What is problematic is control over professional territory, through medical control of the patient and expertise. In the case of the mobility of nurses in intensive care, a highly technical department, it is the question of the expertise required that posed a problem.

In this respect, the experience of two anaesthetists in an operating theatre can be compared.[2] Like others, they testify to the lack of equipment at the start, masks judged to be non-essential by the hierarchy, gowns that are easily torn, and contradictory hygiene instructions. The first wave of COVID was brutal, the operations in the block were cancelled and staff were redeployed to various reanimation services. '*There were plenty of departments to choose from, I was well received, I found colleagues and others who came from the clinics. (...) I was worried beforehand, especially because of the lack of equipment, but afterwards there was good mutual support. We supported each other. It's rare, it worked well, we were all quite motivated, men and women*' (V).

Arriving in another department, C had more mixed feelings, experiencing solidarity limited to 'colleagues who knew each other from the operating theatre', and which was not extended to outsiders in the intensive care unit where she arrived. 'I was not well received and I was not the only one.

---

[2] V has been in the OR for 10 years and C for 20 years. For a long time C alternated between the emergency room and the operating room, but in 2019 he finally chose the OR.

I worked with people I didn't know in the ICU and I found it hard. At the end of the day, the colleagues were eating and they didn't ask us to sit with them. It felt like we were invasive'.

She found herself faced with a divide, in a service 'created from scratch', as she put it, where the local team were 'quite young' and less qualified and found themselves in a situation where they had to be advised by outside contributors, who had more expertise than they did ('There was a lot of equipment they were unfamiliar with. We had to explain things to them'—C). The hierarchy between levels of qualification is a common obstacle to exchanges between colleagues, as the other nurse anaesthetist indirectly testifies. She had a warmer welcome: *'It's true that we specialist nurses don't usually have a good image, and there they appreciated that we mixed with them and we made a contribution, and we talked together. With the orderlies and the hospital care workers it all went well too. (…) We did what we could. I had previous experience of working in pairs'* (V).

In the opposite case, the departmental logic prevailed over mixing (between nomads and sedentary workers). The confrontation of asymmetrical knowledge is delicate. It does not take much ('one or two people') for it to turn sour, for the contribution of outside expertise to be seen as intrusive and for the group to withdraw into itself. In other words, the domination inherent in the medical and paramedical field (Longchamp et al., 2020) is just waiting to resurface. For example, it is important for carers to be greeted by doctors in the department and be called by their first names. By doing so, they bridge the social gap on a daily basis and re-establish a less asymmetrical relationship allowing for interaction (Sainsaulieu, 2007).

Mobilisation in the face of COVID changed the situation. The welcome in the intensive care unit from the doctors was better than that from the carers, according to a pneumology nurse (A), during the second wave. The context was dramatic in October 2020, as staff were told that the wave would be more difficult, and more seriously ill patients were expected. After a short training session ('I had two days of theoretical training, then two days working in tandem with a colleague'), volunteers were placed at the foot of the bed, and the existing staff were afraid that they would have an additional workload by having to train them. *'It lasted a month and a half. I was not badly received but the atmosphere was very heavy. They had been very much impacted. I didn't sense a very good atmosphere. They didn't know where things were going, we didn't talk too much, we had to prove ourselves, they wanted us to help them rather than ask for help. Afterwards they thanked us, but at the beginning they were afraid they would have to train us. They had trained people who didn't want to come back for the second wave. (...) On the other hand, I found their doctors very accessible, the most open. They introduced themselves spontaneously, asking me where I was from. And they thanked us straight away. They were nicer than the carers'* (A).

## 2.3   DOCTORS BETWEEN THE GENERAL AND THE PARTICULAR

Compared to paramedics, doctors are more consistent: they only identify with colleagues, in the department or elsewhere. The only doctors who identify with everyone in the department are the department heads. This leads them on the one hand to defend the general interest of the department, and on the other hand to appropriate 'their' department and 'their' nurses, for better or worse.

In a hierarchical world such as the hospital, denouncing the collective logic of a 'territory' can conceal a class contempt on the part of managers towards less qualified workers or those who rebel against top-down orders. But in practice, hospital managers and doctors have the strongest collective sense, are the most organised and the most separate from the others. They are also the most unionised of all hospital staff: administrative managers are at least three times more unionised than staff (Sainsaulieu, 2008), while doctors have the largest number of unions: in France, they have almost as many unions as there are specialties. So as a group they are closely adapted to their professional territory. The leaders, whether medical or administrative, also have the most personal networks, through which they maintain their positions of power. The trade union is in fact one of the collective resources used as a personal network. Their social capital is reflected in address books which allow them to find help in case of career problems. The difference between carers and managers is not in the geographical distance of relationships. Social capital does not need to be exotic: it only needs to function within a given social space—a field, as Bourdieu would say. So the difference lies more in the number of relationships and in the motivation to solicit them. Indeed, leaders have a career to lead, much more than the people they are leading do. For this purpose, they need elective affinities, good advice and influential contacts. It is the number and quality of relationships that socially distinguish the leader from the led. Apart from that, like their teams, managers pay close attention to what their relations think and can also limit their horizons to better correspond to them, but with greater control over the discourse and the double discourse.

In departments where solidarity is most pronounced, such as the OR, solidarity often extends into private life, and the boundary between professional and private life tends to blur. The block is also known for its 'outings', where everyone meets up to have fun together. Here again, it is an extension of a professional dynamic: to act together, we must know each other well, know how the other will react during an operation, understand each other without words, and not misinterpret behaviour. Knowing each other means getting closer, and getting closer tends to erase the boundaries between the private and the public. Of course, here too people can keep their distance and differentiate between the sexes. But they can also stay together if they want to, and endogamy is a well-known fact of professional socialisation.

In a private clinic in a large city in the west of France, for example, we heard an HR director justify this proximity in a very questionable way. A hospital porter had told us, in the course of a conversation, that he found the nurses in the operating theatre more physically attractive than elsewhere. Although we were sceptical, we repeated this to the HR director, who confirmed this information to us in a personal interview. She made sure that she met the surgeons' expectations in terms of female company. The surgeons were the owners and partners of the clinic.

Is money a motivation for doctors? It is common knowledge that the highest-ranked medical students choose the most recognised and best-paid specialties when they graduate. They do not choose according to the needs of the population. Moreover, professional organisations have always defended their private sector status and refused to allow them to be posted to 'medical deserts' for their first job. Generations of postal workers, on the other hand, have had to wait in Paris for years before being transferred to their home province: they only indicated this by a small flag on a map of France, displayed at the entrance to the 'foyer PTT', the place of residence of postal and telecom employees.

Nothing like that for doctors: they are (left) free and can be hospital employees and freelancers at the same time. They tend to withdraw to the private sector if they can, given the problems encountered in the public hospital. They have varying incomes, with the main divide being between general medicine and hospital medicine, but with huge differences in income within these categories. These incomes are certainly mostly derived from their work, and their personal investment in their work is not solely guided by remuneration. It is safe to say that many see their income as compensation for their work—or do not see it as at all important.

The medical ethos is probably twofold: alongside their professional obligations, which require them to have expert knowledge, doctors oscillate between a universal and a 'bourgeois' morality. On the one hand, medicine is intended for everyone and is based on both a general and a specialised culture. On the other hand, it brings social success and is presented as the guarantee of a privileged social status for people who often come from families in which 'success' is important. In summary, we could say that doctors oscillate between the two poles of universalism and privilege, just as they oscillate between two statuses, that of hospital medicine, based on public service and driving medical research, and that of the private clinic, which is most often profit-oriented and makes it possible to translate accumulated social capital into economic capital. Of course, neither status is unambiguous, and the two are intertwined, to the extent that the clinic can also serve as an adjunct to research and, conversely, since the Debré reform of 1958, the hospital doctor has had a legal percentage of private patients in the public hospital.

## 2.4    CARERS' ROOTS IN THE PEOPLE: CLOSURE OR OPENING?

In France, the reflection on the social rooting of carers refers to a sociology of the working classes. The social hierarchy is reflected in healthcare workers: not only do the lower and higher professional positions in the hospital reproduce the class hierarchy, but this positional hierarchy largely reproduces that of the previous society. In other words, social origins and professional positions most often coincide, and ordinary hospital workers and orderlies do not come from the same social background as doctors. Basically, we find the three-way split between the working classes, middle classes and upper classes in the healthcare hierarchy. The qualifications of nurses place them in their majority in the middle classes, but their social origin clearly divides them into two blocks: those from the working classes and those from the middle classes. Hence the ambiguity of their positions.

For example, nurses sometimes see themselves as mere employees and sometimes as privileged assistants to doctors. Few nurses in France see themselves solely as nurses. They tend to lean one way or the other.

Qualitatively, this is reflected in the interviews, in their position in relation to strikes or the social world, and in their ability to leave the hospital to work as independent nurses, to retrain or to give up work altogether. This can be seen indirectly in their votes in professional elections: the nurses' unions have very few votes in France. Nurses either vote for the general salaried unions or do not vote at all. Overall they vote less than non-healthcare workers in hospitals, while care assistants tend to vote more and to organise more than nurses in the general confederal unions.

The position of carers in relation to the COVID vaccine underlines this social hierarchy: the higher up carers were in the professional hierarchy, the more quickly they were vaccinated. In other words, working-class people were the most reluctant to be vaccinated, including among healthcare workers. Why was this?

A recent study provides some answers for the French population overall. The study compared the '*prevalence of vaccination reluctance in general and COVID-19 vaccine hesitancy and social and health factors associated with intentions to receive the vaccine*' (Bajos et al., 2022). It found that '*people at the bottom of the social hierarchy, in terms of level of education and financial resources, were more likely to refuse the COVID-19 vaccine*'. In addition, two other significant results showed that '*people from the French overseas departments, immigrants and descendants of immigrants, were all more reluctant to have the COVID-19 vaccine*' and that '*those who reported not trusting the government were more likely to be COVID-19 vaccine-reluctant*'. Vaccine reluctance preceded the pandemic: in 2015, the French were already much less favourable to the flu vaccine (52% in favour) than their British or Spanish neighbours (85% and 80%). The study on COVID vaccine resistance showed strong continuity in this intra-European contrast. The social gap is even widening in France: '*the lower they were in the social hierarchy, the more reluctant people were to be vaccinated in general and to have the COVID-19 vaccine in particular*'. The reluctant population was also more female, younger and more 'racialised' ('those from the overseas departments [DOM], immigrants and descendants of immigrants from Africa/Asia'). And also more defiant towards the government.

How should we interpret these results? There is no simple hypothesis.

The idea that populations living far from urban centres or from reliable sources of information are underinformed, particularly for the elderly, has as its corollary, particularly for young people, in a greater permeability to the fake news circulating on social networks. So in this hypothesis, under-information and disinformation converge.

Next, the question of politicisation is to be considered but also in a dual way: not only the politics of protest, which leads to the rejection of everything that comes from the government, but also an alternative politicisation. Atypical convictions (religious, naturalistic, bioethical, etc.) would in this sense lead to a relativisation of science, progress or medicine. Nevertheless, the above-mentioned survey shows a high rate of support for science (80%, twice as high as confidence in the political authorities). It would, therefore, be necessary to verify whether people who refuse vaccinations have less confidence in science and medicine.

The politicisation of protest seems to be more established by previous surveys. The cited paper showed that trust in government was 'the variable with the strongest effect' on reluctance to vaccinate against COVID-19, even more than for vaccines in general. '*In a country such as France, public authorities have close control over the supply and marketing of vaccines. So, people's propensity to trust the government, the leading actor in the country's vaccination strategy, has affected attitudes toward vaccination. The French government has been harshly criticised for failing to anticipate the crisis and for wanting to cover up the lack of masks, claiming until April 2020 that they were not necessary to protect people from the virus*'. In support of this thesis, one could think of a continuity of protest between social movements, from the Yellow Vests to the anti-vax and/or anti-pass demonstrations. But it is not certain that the demonstrators were the same in the two periods of agitation: according to the testimony of an activist who attended both types of demonstration in Besançon (eastern France), the two audiences were very different. It would, therefore, be necessary to study the protest content and its continuities/discontinuities, particularly in the care sector.

Some hypotheses focus on social groups. Thus the prevalence of women in criticising vaccines, particularly concerning children, suggests a different relationship to the body. Female control of the body, family planning and the domestic space, via preventive nutritional practices, would be threatened in the eyes of some women by the medical control embodied by the vaccine. Similarly, African-American ethnic-racial minorities in the US are more likely to reject vaccines: '*Numerous studies have shown that ethno-racial minorities have less confidence in the healthcare system and in caregivers than the majority population*'. As a result, the authors suggest the need to reconsider the vaccination strategy used in France ('based exclusively on epidemiological criteria') by focusing on some groups which are harder to convince than others in the vaccination campaign: '*women, youth, the working class, ethno-racial minorities*'.

If we turn to caregivers, we see the following paradox: while they are more able to understand the urgency of the vaccination campaign, they are also more likely to mistrust the government which did not establish good conditions to face the pandemic. We can also imagine that rank-and-file employees were most exposed to the pandemic. In other words, the workers paid a higher price for bad working conditions than doctors.

Traditionally, the trade union has sought to overcome contradictions in the workforce. However, it is not immune to contradictions either, particularly in the care sector.

## BIBLIOGRAPHY

Bajos, N., Spire, A., Silberzan, L., & for the EPICOV Study Group. (2022). The Social Specificities of Hostility Toward Vaccination against Covid-19 in France. *PLoS ONE, 17*(1), e0262192. https://doi.org/10.1371/journal.pone.0262192

Castra, M., & Sainsaulieu, I. (2020). Intervenir sur un autre territoire professionnel. Equipes mobiles et services sédentaires à l'hôpital. *Sciences sociales et santé, 38*(4), 47–74.

Longchamp, P., Toffel, K., Bühlmann, F., & Tawfik, A. (2020). *L'espace infirmier. Visions et divisions d'une profession.* Livreo-Alphil, Neuchâtel, 258.

Sainsaulieu, I. (2007). *L'hôpital et ses acteurs. Appartenances et égalité.* Belin, Perspectives sociologiques.

Sainsaulieu, I. (2008). Le syndicalisme à l'hôpital. Sociologie d'une insatisfaction. Dossier Syndicalisme et santé, *Les Tribunes de la santé*, n°18, 83–94.

Sainsaulieu, I. (2009). Le bon patient est sous contrôle. Communautés de service et pratiques soignantes à l'hôpital. *Revue suisse de sociologie – Swiss Journal of Sociology, 35*(3), 551–570.

# CHAPTER 3

# Institutional Trade Unionism

**Abstract** It is neither possible nor desirable to leave trade unionism aside when addressing the issue of work collectives. Of course, the hospital is not the most important place for trade unionism, particularly in France, where nurses are a rare commodity in union sections. But the limit is not only sectoral, it is also structural and results from the bureaucratisation of trade unionism. We return to the paradox of this union bureaucracy, which is both stable and unstable, like the bureaucracy in general, before sketching out a comparative periodisation between France and the US. We then leave the literature to show concretely how the split operates between employees and trade unions in the example of the banking sector, to conclude on the hospital sector.

**Keywords** Unions • Healthcare militants • Union bureaucracy • Union bases

In France, trade unionism today is based on a structural misunderstanding which confuses the capacity for collective action of employees, a minority of activists and a trade union apparatus. This misunderstanding, which is often deliberate, makes it possible to emphasise one or other factor, depending on the political orientation adopted and the audience addressed.

Born of the collective movement, trade unionism represents it. This discrepancy finds its traditional legitimacy in the mechanism of

© The Author(s), under exclusive license to Springer Nature
Singapore Pte Ltd. 2023
I. Sainsaulieu, *Care Staff Mobilisation in the Hospital*,
https://doi.org/10.1007/978-981-19-9354-1_3

31

representation, asserted since the English Revolution and reaffirmed by the French Revolution, during which the deputies renounced any imperative mandate very early on and during which national sovereignty replaced popular sovereignty (Tackett, 1997). It is also rooted in a militant tradition that generates inequality of investment in the collective: depending on age, experience, training and involvement in the workplace, people are more or less committed to defending a cause. Thus, active minorities defend the others or prepare the ground for broader actions. This is the theme of the avant-garde, which is very much present in international trade unionism, through the anarchist and communist currents that historically inhabited it, as trade unionism emerged and developed in the early twentieth century. In France, in a more pragmatic context, radical syndicalism resurfaced in the 1990s (Sainsaulieu, 1999; Lequeux & Sainsaulieu, 2010).

But if these avant-garde activists are distinguished by deeply held convictions, they also risk cutting themselves off from the working population by gaining access to delegation hours which free them from ordinary activity. Especially since, while it is possible to continue devoting oneself to others while being a delegate, one can also be attracted from the outset by the material situation of a union official. Finally, the political orientation followed by the union highlights this or that aspect at a particular time and creates a precedent for the future. Thus, the theme of the bureaucratisation of trade unionism is as old as the latter, sometimes from the point of view of the formation of a foreign social body with its own interests, and sometimes as an institutional representative of the interests of the ruling class.

## 3.1    What Is Bureaucracy? Back to the Classics

The discussion on trade union bureaucratisation has its roots in the theory of bureaucracy. In *Economy and Society*, Max Weber characterises bureaucracy as a rational hierarchical principle, setting administrative rules. He defines the notion of bureaucracy as an administrative structure based on well-defined and hierarchical offices and functions. However, the question of the advent of bureaucracy is not central to his thinking. We know that for him there is a size effect, a threshold beyond which the organisation becomes more complex and necessarily bureaucratic. We also know that at the macro-social level, the spirit of capitalism is the bearer of bureaucratic rationality. Rational modernisation is bureaucratic and compatible with the capitalist economy, if not carried by it. Whereas Marx stigmatised the 'anarchy' of the process of capitalist accumulation, Max Weber sees it as a process of rationalisation.

As a result, Max Weber's teleology is based on a perennial or even expanding bureaucracy, while Marx's teleology only sees bureaucracy as a temporary outgrowth of the history of the class struggle. Thus, Louis Napoleon Bonaparte's coup d'état of 18 Brumaire 1851 consecrates the advent of a 'parasitic body' above society, at a post-revolutionary moment of exhaustion of the 'historical' social classes, the bourgeoisie and the proletariat. In contrast, for Marx, the peasantry, a composite group without coherence like a sack of potatoes, favours the emergence of state leaders with no other role than to give life to a strange structure, a disproportionate state as if suspended above society: 'The state seems to have made itself independent of society, to have subjugated it' (Marx, 1852–2014).

This approach is taken up and extended by Trotsky to explain the weight of the state in the so-called semi-Bonapartist regimes, characterised by the weakness of the national bourgeoisie and the weight of foreign capital: 'The governments of backward, i.e., colonial and semi-colonial countries, by and large assume a Bonapartist or semi-Bonapartist character; and differ from one another in this, that some try to move in a democratic direction, seeking support among workers and peasants, while others install a form close to military-police dictatorship' (Trotsky, 1940). In this view, bureaucracy vacillates between a stable and unstable character. It does have a structural side, since it derives from the nature of entire societies, but these societies are on the fringe of the historical matrix, of the capitalist machine that feeds the economic, social and political revolution. The fate of these peripheral societies depends on the countries where modern social classes clash. The USSR was typical of this characterisation as a by-product of a titanic struggle, as the runt of the world revolution. Trotsky even compared the Soviet bureaucracy to a 'marble on top of a pyramid', to underline its instability, linked to its parasitic character. The Soviet bureaucracy did eventually tip over to one side, to the market, by appropriating and dismantling the state economy with the rapacity of parvenus, who were soon transformed into oligarchs.

But the duration of her prior Soviet reign fuelled a pained debate among Trotskyists about the 'nature of the USSR', about whether a 'bureaucratic society' existed, as theorised by Cornelius Castoriadis (Raynaud, 1989). For Castoriadis, 'state capitalism' corresponded to a lasting domination in a new type of unequal society. The 'Asian mode of production' (AMP) represents another attempt to describe a society where the state plays a structural role, following Marx and Engels' remarks about an 'Asian mode of production' where the state 'replaced' the bourgeoisie in the organisation of society. The AMP theoretically underpins a multi-secular social formation characterised by the intertwining of the state and traditional peasant communities (Dhoquois, 1966).

In contrast, more recent writings on neoliberal bureaucratisation emphasise the dependence of the state on exogenous social domination. David Graeber is the most explicit: if a 'timorous spirit', and therefore bureaucracy, has invaded even the social sciences, it is because capitalism has renounced technological progress in favour of a conservative domination favourable to finance (Graeber, 2015). This is the profound meaning of the multiplication of controls: by curbing technology, oligopolistic and financial capitalism has moved away from 'creative technologies' towards the 'bureaucratic technologies' of surveillance, labour, discipline and administrative tasks. Administrative imperatives have thus become political ends in themselves, not technical means. But the bureaucracy has not become independent of the social and economic elite, to which it is closely linked. The example of the birth of the German social state is significant for him: Bismarck explicitly created a social bureaucracy to prevent the labour movement from establishing social and democratic control. In doing so, he created a matrix from which later socialist governments also drew (Graeber, 2015, p. 181). Bureaucracy has a tendency to persevere in its being, even resisting the efforts of progressive rulers, but it is not a substitute for social domination.

In contrast to the apostles of the critique of totalitarianism, from whom she distances herself, Béatrice Hibou also defends (what I call) a 'dependentist' perspective on bureaucracy, due to superior socio-economic interests. She emphasises the classical attachment of Marx and Weber to social domination: for Weber, 'the being of the bureaucracy lay in its subordination to its masters' (Hibou, 2012, p. 110), even though, in his view, the bureaucracy could accommodate 'any dominant interest' (ibid.). Similarly, current formalisation procedures have multiplied to meet socio-economic needs of 'delocalisation, subcontracting, decomposition of production processes and fragmentation of the value chain' (idem, p. 116). This material process of global reordering of capitalism leads to a need for homogenisation through an 'explosion of norms', standardisation, procedures, controls and audits that constitute the 'invisible chains' of domination' (ibid.).

However, it is not so simple to establish a univocal dependency perspective, because bureaucratisation is not a simple transmission belt. For David Graeber, bureaucracy has a strong legitimacy, due to the social need for impersonal logics and ambivalent rules, which are both constraining and regulating. For Beatrice Hibou, bureaucratisation remains partly indeterminate and elusive through its capacity to generate a 'bureaucratic participation' of actors: experts, consultants and managers form the network and the social base of the bureaucracy, its first circles. But the rational legitimacy with which bureaucracy drapes itself finds a wider echo: today, as in the past, the dominant and the dominated can each demand rational control for themselves, with bureaucracy-mixing formalities and collective expectations, just as individuals are both victims and actors of neoliberalism, all the more so since the neoliberal bureaucracy is characterised less by 'institutional and administrative characteristics' than by 'abstract formalities' covering 'a constellation of heterogeneous interests' (Hibou, 2012, p. 152). The result is a multi-dimensional and flexible 'bureaucratic labyrinth', where informalities and formalities intersect, and 'which shapes domination in the power relations, conflicts and arrangements it gives rise to' (idem., p. 189).

In short, bureaucracy is sometimes an independent, self-sustaining phenomenon, and sometimes a dependent phenomenon, closely linked to an exogenous social domination. However, its social anchorage legitimises domination, from below as well as from above. Marx and Weber converge in their own way on this point, since for Weber the rational-legal legitimacy of bureaucracy makes it widely acceptable, while Marx condemns its parasitism, but nevertheless anchors it socially: the social basis of the Bonapartist bureaucratic regime is the peasantry, but it is also a social compromise between the historical classes, due to their inability to prevail. However transient and super-structural it may be, it also has a social and political raison d'être.

So, we can conclude that bureaucracy is probably too complex a social phenomenon to be explained in a single way. It has multiple facets depending on the angle, place and time considered. It can be broken down into different elements (administrative, political, economic, social, technological, institutional, normative, elitist, participatory, rational, parasitic, material and immaterial, etc.), which change in meaning depending on the historical context. In recent times, bureaucracy has taken the form of procedures rather than institutions, very much subservient to the competitive market and/or to monopolistic capitalism, financial rather than productive, conservative rather than progressive.

These classical and modern debates have the merit of underlining the ambivalence attached to the theoretical definition of bureaucracy, which is more or less stable, independent and durable depending on the perspectives given. Is it a cork to be popped or a lasting institution? Analyses of trade union bureaucracy also highlight both endogenous and exogenous factors.

## 3.2    THE FACES OF INSTITUTIONALISATION IN FRANCE AND THE US

The institutionalisation of trade unionism is a quasi-generic problem, since the existence of illegal trade unions was gradually replaced by the standard of legalisation which became widespread in industrial countries at the end of the nineteenth century. Criticism of the benefits of legality was, however, voiced by the actors themselves from the outset (Mouriaux, 2006). The academic debate echoed this through the 'iron law of oligarchy' of Robert Michels (1911–2015), a pupil of Max Weber, for whom leaders tend to professionalise and then monopolise power at the same time as changing their outlook, abandoning their idealism and becoming sceptical. However, political parties have been the subject of more developed sociological criticism than trade unions, especially in France. Motsei Ostrogorski's pioneering critique (1912) highlighted the dispossession of citizens by the partisan body, which elaborated its programmes without their knowledge and abused party patriotism to prevent any criticism, or even to favour clientelist practices (Cazes, 1993). In Ostrogorski's view, parties, once in power, depoliticise the debate by favouring their adaptation to the majority of the electorate and the technical implementation of laws. He thus inaugurated a critique of the professionalisation of parties and the disconnect between the logic of representation and citizens' control, and even made a plea for direct democracy in favour of temporary parties focused on a specific issue.

From a historical perspective, several logics of institutionalisation have followed one another and intertwined (Sainsaulieu, 2017).

The first logic is ideological: it is the adherence to political values that guides trade union action. As soon as it is legally recognised, trade unionism must respect the foundations of the French Republic and, in particular, the sacrosanct private property of the companies in which it operates. At the same time, after unification within the CGT, trade unionism proclaimed its membership of a revolutionary current (whose principles were adopted in the Amiens Charter, named after the venue for the CGT congress in 1906), and this identity was reinforced by its allegiance to communism. This allegiance followed the ups and downs of the international communist movement but did not waver in the second twentieth century, with the defence of the revolution becoming a defence of the USSR. Whether it was a question of adherence to the Republic, the revolution or the USSR, this political priority imposed itself on the trade union agenda, including, and above all, in terms of strikes, which were launched or curbed not only according to the potential for social protest to advance the wage-workers' cause but first and foremost according to this political priority.

A second logic is that of bureaucratic inflation. Its premises lie in a social differentiation within the proletariat. As early as 1858, Engels criticised the gentrification of part of the English workers. Marx and then Bakunin criticised the social integration of the 'workers' aristocracy', the upper layers of the wage-earners who enjoyed a privileged social status. The phenomenon continues to this day, with strata of employees differentiating themselves by gaining access to advantages due to their working conditions and their strategic socio-economic position: train drivers in France are called 'rail barons', while air traffic controllers, employees of the Bank of France or EDF electricians have also obtained statutory advantages that are important for employees and useful for social peace. Not forgetting civil servants, who make up for their modest remuneration with benefits in kind, due to the strength of their numbers—the state being the largest employer in France since the Second World War.

On the organisational level, permanent trade union officials appeared as trade union rights were extended, due to the strength of the labour movement, particularly in these bastions. Trade union 'permanency' became necessary to keep the institutions of social dialogue alive. It grew to considerable proportions during the Thirty Glorious Years due to the rate of economic growth, the size of the working class and the development of paritarianism (Unedic, Social Security, etc.). It reached its peak with the creation of union delegates after May 1968. These appointed delegates had the task of controlling elected staff delegates. Similarly, the management of lifelong learning, created in 1972, was partly entrusted to the trade unions.

As the classic analyses of bureaucracy suggest, this bureaucratic trade union force nurtures a social compromise that benefits both employees and employers, within the framework of a given balance of power. If in the first period the trade union bureaucracy controlled the employees in exchange for social reforms, the period that began at the end of the 1970s changed the situation.

A third logic is that of bureaucratic deflation. As the de-industrialisation of jobs in France began (more than the bankruptcy of French industrial groups, which concentrated and redeployed their lucrative activities internationally), the number of workers, union members and strikes fell from the mid-1970s onwards. This spiral movement has continued throughout the 'unhappy thirty years' until the present day, even if the pace fluctuated from one decade to the next. The result was a weakening of trade unionism, whose head swelled disproportionately to its body. In a trend of affirmation of the power of capital, the unions have seen a triple evolution: firstly, legislation ended up correcting their representativeness, by questioning the reality of their establishment. Secondly, the line of trade unionism was moderated, with the refocusing of main unions, the CFDT, CGT and FO in the 1980s and 1990s—with the end of the USSR as an additional moment of this political détente. Lastly, a logic of 'between ourselves' developed as never before in management circles, with confederal officials being as if bewitched by the triumphant figure of the boss, as well as human resources managers (Surdez et al., 2018). Repeated scandals in recent years have demonstrated the strength of this strange attraction in the main trade unions, with a series of embezzlements of public funds for private use (CGT), transfers of former leaders to the private sector (CFDT) or pantagruelian expense accounts of leading members (FO).

In the US, the bureaucratisation of trade unionism is well documented. The significance of this has been equally ambivalent since the Second World War: colleagues describe the rise of unionisation and a union power favourable to employees, on the one hand, and the emergence of a force independent of employees and close to employers, on the other.

The first point of view is illustrated by S. M. Jacoby (2004). At the end of the Second World War, a transformation had taken place, to the benefit of workers. Union pressure had succeeded in converting millions of day-to-day jobs into sustainable ones, at the expense of the flexibility of the labour market. The spread of protected internal labour markets was replacing an open society. In the political arena, where they had become a powerful force, unions sought to expand programmes—national unemployment insurance, higher minimum wages, full employment laws—to increase the gains already achieved through collective bargaining. In the workplace, union members were protected by a variety of job security schemes that mimicked other companies. It was these 'rigidities', described as a 'new industrial feudalism', that neoliberal currents later sought to challenge.

In the other narrative, bureaucratisation has a less worker-friendly face (Fantasia & Voss, 2003). The association of trade unions with the war effort during the Second World War and the subsequent movement towards bureaucratisation led to a post-war 'button-press unionism' that was the antithesis of the 'spontaneity of trade unionism in previous decades'. Pioneering activists, or those most active in the field, were pushed aside in favour of specialised managers (negotiators, managers, civil servants, lawyers). The automatic deduction of dues increased the gap with the field, weakening the link between solidarity at work and union solidarity and transforming the relationship with the union into one of a service provider. Business agents replaced organisers, managing existing union agreements and the growing standard of dispute resolution, while the leaders of the big unions increasingly resembled the business leaders themselves: they too sat on company boards but were more smooth-talking, conformist and discreet than other leaders, looking like junior, loyal and obedient managers. The head of the big American union (AFL-CIO), Kirkland, unknown to union members when he took over the leadership, remained unknown to the general public when he retired in 1998, 16 years later. Other leaders were and still are autocrats, because of their undemocratic methods of operation, some going so far as to confuse union funds with their own funds for personal enrichment, in connection with the mafia circles that the authorities mobilised during the Second World War or afterwards to strike against the strikers, in the docks of New York (and Marseille).

## 3.3 Two Trade Union Bases. The Example of the Banking Sector

We have investigated the distance between the 'base' and the top of the trade union hierarchy. In a survey of the banking sector in France, which used two questionnaires to question union members of a bank on the one hand and members of the CGT banking federation on the other, we found elements of dissociation (Sainsaulieu, 2014). In the monographic questionnaire on the bank, it is not so much the employees who reject the CGT (41% of respondents do not want to join) as the CGT which does not invite them to meetings (according to 71% of respondents). On the one hand, people do not feel invited, while on the other, they willingly judge bank employees as 'individualistic': there is indeed a discrepancy.

Moreover, the two lines of the trade union are partially contradicted: social dialogue is accepted without enthusiasm (or even without illusions), the respondents having little knowledge of the agreements concluded by their trade union; social criticism does not lead to combativeness (strikes are notoriously excluded from the possibilities of action).

As it stands, this material shows support for trade unionism as a moral principle, for the defence of employees, beyond the knowledge of its limits. Trade unionism is still perceived as a protective shield in the event of a hard blow, but the link is loose between its internal components (union leadership, activists, members) and its socio-professional environment. So it also shows the limits of militancy, not supported as in the past by compact homogeneous groups, but threatened on the contrary with delegitimisation by members with different emphases, including on the core of the class convictions dear to the organisation.

The survey was an opportunity to make the notion of the union base more complex. The CGT's unionised milieu has always been influenced by the union's (or the party's) line, and the state of mind of the employees has not always been a determining factor in that line. The difference with the current situation seems to us twofold: on the one hand, it is not so much the line as the divisions, the tensions which now permeate downwards; on the other hand, it is not so much the CGT union members in the strict sense who respond, as a distinct, homogeneous (and thick) layer, but rather a composite company milieu, made up of CGT members and other unions, non-members and permanent or occasional CGT voters. The milieu of union members is less important than it once was, and militants have become used to evolving in a subjectively circumscribed company milieu (according to their criteria and their relations), rather than aiming first and foremost at the objectively defined 'insiders'—except for electoral issues.

A certain discrepancy is perceptible between the concerns of the two bases, the company environment and the unionised environment, just as a marked left-wing politicisation seems to distinguish the former militants of the federation from more recent members.

Within the trade union population responding to the federal interbank questionnaire, a clear contrast appears between recent members and militants. A very political and committed hard core of militants from the 1968 generation stand out, advocating harder positions and a strong CGT identity. We also know that these militants, who are few in number, are very attached to the union and largely keep it alive. Thus, the pre-2000 members formed a more politicised group, with more mandates. They are more attached and loyal to the CGT, having tried fewer other unions and are prouder to belong to it. These members have more members and a greater sense of their duties as union members towards the union.

In the face of this radical loyalty, the categories of female, younger and more recent members show a certain autonomy of judgement on the part of employees in relation to the union, concerning the professional content to be given to work (as opposed to the working environment) and the specific deterioration of working conditions (and no longer with a workerist ideological prism). Another, xenophobic sensibility, of distrust of the 'number of immigrants', especially concerns recent members. Newer members have known the CGT more through the media and want to devote less time to it and take on fewer internal or Works Council responsibilities. Their commitment is more oriented towards the employees than towards the organisation. They are just as much involved in a work collective but are more critical of the way the union works in terms of the efforts to involve union members and employees, while they exonerate the union members themselves from criticism. They also have slightly less confidence in the union's word. The gap is noticeable with regard to politics. 'Recent' members are less keen on anything that has a political connotation or broad, societal concerns: international solidarity, the Arab revolution (they are even slightly more xenophobic, with 7 percentage points more positive responses to the question: 'What do you think of the statement: there are too many immigrants in France? Agree, disagree?').

We noted difficulties in legitimising both moderate and radical trade union strategies. In this context, we understand how militants favouring protest can maintain their cause because of the difficulties felt by the employees close to them (workload and working conditions), but we see employees, whether or not they are members of the union, expressing a certain moderation and a wide range of concerns (bonuses, mobility, interest in the job). In particular, the identity aspects of work are expressed by employees, especially by managers and young people for whom union activity can be a 'means of identity and cultural expression' to compensate for the loss of job. It should be noted that this contrast in politicisation between the generations is not uniform and changes according to the context: in Chile, for example, a new post-dictatorship generation has been able to claim greater politicisation of the CUT trade union centre (Guttierez-Crocco, 2012).

In France, the dividing line is not so much between the rank and file and the union leadership as between the militants and the recent members, who do not feel represented, invest little in trade unionism or rely on experienced militants to drive union activity. We can, therefore, reassess the division between moderate and radical militants. If the position of leader encourages moderation and the position of opponent encourages radicalism, the opinions are not always different. Both come from the same socialisation at work and/or have experienced more or less the same politicisation software—both generational and organisational, for the most part from the French Communist Party, as we observed in meetings and interviews.

The reflection on the existence of the base also allows us to find a junction between top-down internal functioning and bottom-up employee sentiment. The legitimacy of the central leaders is not only diminished by the fact that their competence is equal to that of their challengers in the union fiefdoms, but also by the fact that it is not sanctified, supported or stabilised by the presence of a strong participation.

## 3.4   Limits of Trade Unionism in Hospitals

Employee trade unionism, which originated with the workers, has had difficulty adapting to the hospital. White coats have long since replaced blue collars, and the number of doctors has only increased. The hospital was once a small world of its own, with its workers, technicians, boiler room staff, laundry, kitchen and hospital staff. Since 1945, it has been professionalised in stages, medicalised and refocused on its professions (Sainsaulieu, 2007). Like airports, it has become a model of standardised professional bureaucracy throughout the world, including in countries of the South, such as Senegal, where a few large cities, notably the capital Dakar, have a healthcare provision out of all proportion to rural and semi-urban regions (Diallo & Sainsaulieu, 2022).

This highly technical and professional world does not necessarily play into the hands of employee unions. Thus, while doctors' unions are numerous in France and nurses' unions have remained insignificant, nurses have kept their distance from the inter-category trade unionism represented in France notably by the CGT (*Confédération Générale du Travail,* 1898), the CFDT (*Confédération Française Démocratique du Travail,* 1964), FO (*Force Ouvrière,* 1947) and, since the 1990s, *Sud Santé-Socials* (a member of Solidaires) and the UNSA (*Union Nationale des Syndicats Autonomes*).

None of the unions has recorded a significant increase in membership or activists for decades. The membership rate remains structurally low (12% in the public sector, less than 8% in the private sector), without comparison with the 'real bastions' of the public sector, even if they are in decline, such as the national education system, SNCF railway workers or EDF electricians, and not much higher than the national average (7%). The unions themselves complain about a certain disconnection. They deplore the rate of electoral abstention, which is particularly high among paramedics, reaching 50% at the turn of the century, according to Sud Santé (Solidaires). The CGT and especially FO are not well established among nurses (there are no statistics on the number of union members per profession). The Solidaires union also deplores 'the low level of consideration' for these care professions, all unions combined, while the CFDT notes 'a withdrawal of care workers from the confederated unions' (Sainsaulieu, 2008a).

Studies have been carried out by this organisation. As a result of the negative image of trade unionism in general, the CFDT appears ambivalent, with a gap between announcements and achievements (Visier, 1992). It has difficulty justifying its action locally, and even adopts a low profile. However, legibility is all the more necessary in large establishments, where relations between employees and trade unions are looser, and where the role of trade unionism as a social agency tends to take precedence over the role of leader or mediator of the social movement. Solidaires notes that progress in terms of membership is mainly in small structures, particularly medico-social ones, where an activist can have a stronger influence than in the large segmented hospitals, in connection with the establishment in the department.

Trade unionists are not satisfied with this situation of withdrawal into a relationship between voters and elected representatives. There is even a guilt complex on the part of the militants, an 'unhappy conscience' in the face of such recognition without trust on the part of the employees. Nor have the employees resigned themselves to this 'exteriority'. They have vague and contradictory demands: they ask for information closer to their activity and, at the same time, the trade union is called upon (like the management) to play the role of referee in the relations between employees from different categories or departments (Vincent & Volovitch, 2002).

The employees recognise the usefulness of an institutional role, but this role prevents them from experiencing a feeling of belonging that would produce confidence. On the contrary, the so-called coordinations make use of the feeling of proximity, of identity, even of collective fusion, without their institutional role being very well recognised (belonging to a 'group in fusion' is temporary). The unions do not enter into work practices and remain outside the practical issues of work organisation. Local managers seem to compensate for the union deficit by emphasising participation and mobilisation for the quality of care. Although they tend to exaggerate the scope of participatory mechanisms, as nurses are much less enthusiastic and generally do not spare P&MS from criticism, the teams find that P&MS play a rather useful role and rely on them to solve the problems of the 'collective'. P&MS reciprocate, as they want to be recognised as a priority by the staff and feel little consulted by their management (Sainsaulieu, 2008b). The distant trade unions are matched by 'active' P&MS. The unions, for their part, attest to the participation of nurses in committees to improve the quality of care.

A monograph helps us to appreciate the situation in the health sector in the US and to better highlight the gap between unionism and healthcare workers (Reich, 2012). For the author, the ethical dimension of care must be more strongly supported by the union, in a context of moral overkill by management. Studying the case of a private Catholic clinic, he considers that the values of healthcare should not be the prerogative of the management's discourse and that the union cannot be satisfied with economic demands and power relations in this context. Caregivers are loyal to the institution as an establishment serving the community. As is the case in small private clinics in France, nurses are attached to their colleagues and do not consider leaving for better pay elsewhere. More generally, the author suggests that the classic opposing strategies of voice and loyalty are not so relevant in a context of care which insists on its professional and ethical dimension.

In summary, the gap between trade unionism and employees is not new. In France, it has a rich history, made up of various periods and factors. Nevertheless, this gap is expressed a little differently in hospitals among healthcare workers. It is true that the unionised environment (the union base) is much smaller than the business environment (hospital employees). But it is also confronted with the separation between carers and non-carers (not to mention the separation between doctors and paramedics: doctors have specific unions, based on medical specialities or even sub-specialities). The trade unionism of all hospital staff is both more working class and less 'basist' than that of the care workers. It represents non-care workers better than care workers, which means that there is a first gap, since the majority of hospital employees are care workers. Similarly, its presence among female nurses is more noticeable among orderlies than among nurses, although the nursing corps is larger than that of orderlies. But alongside these quantitative discrepancies, there is a qualitative discrepancy: the unions do not follow the moods of care workers. We will come back to this later. Before doing so, we need to explore the significance of the sectoral mobilisation of care workers.

## BIBLIOGRAPHY

Cazes, B. (1993). *Motsei Ostrogorski. La démocratie et les partis politiques.* In *Politique étrangère,* n°2, 58ᶜannée, 516–517.

Dhoquois, G. (1966). Le mode de production asiatique. *Cahiers Internationaux de Sociologie, 41,* 83–92. http://www.jstor.org/stable/40689370

Diallo, A. M., & Sainsaulieu, I. (2022). Les agents de « santé communautaire » au Sénégal. Unité et segmentation d'un groupe semi-professionnel en milieu rural et péri-urbain. *Sciences sociales et santé, 40,* 5–28.

Fantasia, R., & Voss, K. (2003). *Des syndicats domestiqués.* Répression patronale et résistance syndicale aux États-Unis. Raisons d'agir.

Graeber, D. (2015). *Bureaucratie, l'utopie des règles.* Les liens qui libèrent.

Guttierez-Crocco, F. (2012). Les archipels militants dans le syndicalisme chilien ou la frontière revisitée entre syndicalisme et politique. In I. Sainsaulieu & M. Surdez (Dir.), *Sens politiques du travail.* Armand Colin, coll. "Recherche".

Hibou, B. (2012). *La bureaucratisation du monde à l'ère néolibérale.* La Découverte.

Jacoby, S. M. (2004). *Employing Bureaucracy.* Taylor & Francis Group.

Lequeux, S., & Sainsaulieu, I. (2010). Social Movement Unionism in France: A Case for Revitalisation? *Labor Studies Journal, 35*(4), 503–519.

Mouriaux, R. (2006). Syndicalisme et politique: liaison dangereuse ou tragédie moderne? *Mouvements, 43*(1), 30–35.

Ostrogorski, M. (1912). *La démocratie et les partis politiques.* Calmann-Lévy.

Raynaud, P. (1989). Société bureaucratique et totalitarisme. Remarques sur l'évolution du groupe 'Socialisme ou Barbarie'. In G. Busino (Ed.), *Autonomie et autotransformation de la société. La philosophie militante de Cornelius Castoriadis* (pp. 255–268). Librairie Droz.

Reich, A. D. (2012). *With God on Our Side: The Struggle for Workers' Rights in a Catholic Hospital.* Cornell University Press.

Sainsaulieu, I. (1999). Sud-PTT: A Political Trade Unionism? *Industrial Relations, 54*(4), 790–814.

Sainsaulieu, I. (2007). *L'hôpital et ses acteurs. Appartenances et égalité.* Belin, Perspectives sociologiques.

Sainsaulieu, I. (2008a). Le syndicalisme à l'hôpital. Sociologie d'une insatisfaction. Dossier Syndicalisme et santé, *Les Tribunes de la santé*, n°18, 83–94.

Sainsaulieu, I. (2008b). Le cadre animateur: figure fragile d'une conciliation légitime. In I. Sainsaulieu (Dir.), *Les cadres hospitaliers. Représentations et pratiques.* Lamarre.

Sainsaulieu, I. (2014). Retour sur la notion de 'base syndicale'. Le milieu de la CGT des banques en tensions. *L'Homme et la Société*, n°193–194, juin–décembre, 13–41.

Sainsaulieu, I. (2017). *Conflits et résistances au travail* (p. 150). SciencesPo Les Presses, coll. "Conteser".

Surdez, M., Zufferey, E., Sainsaulieu, I., Plomb, F., & Poglia Mileti, F. (2018). *L'enracinement professionnel des opinions politiques. Enquête auprès d'agriculteurs, d'ingénieurs et de directeurs de ressources humaines exerçant en Suisse.* Seismo.

Tackett, T. (1997). *Par la volonté du peuple. Comment les députés de 1789 sont devenus révolutionnaires.* Albin Michel.

Trotsky, L. (1940). *Les syndicats à l'époque de la décadence impérialiste.* Brochure.

Vincent, C., & Volovitch, P. (2002). *Les syndicats face aux restructurations hospitalières: entre défense des personnels et gestion des systèmes de santé.* Institut de Recherche et d'Etudes sur le Syndicalisme.

Visier, L. (1992). L'image des syndicats dans les gros établissements hospitaliers. Confédération Française Démocratique du Travail.

# CHAPTER 4

# Alternative Models of Caring and Hesitant Practices

**Abstract** Is there an alternative model to the exhausting work of carers? For a while, we believed in the advent of a service society where the patient, like the user, would be at the heart of the work. We were disappointed: neither the rise of the tertiary sector nor that of high technology or digital technology in themselves guarantee a better society. The meaning of care work is itself under debate. Sometimes it is given a feminist meaning, insofar as it carries a concrete morality, sometimes it has as its corollary the reproduction of male domination and the sacrifice of women. Moreover, attempts to promote more inclusive and patient-friendly practices always come up against the same hierarchical obstacles.

**Keywords** Care society • Care work • Feminism • Alternative care practices

A second frequent reflection on the caregiving 'vocation' is the opposite of the first. Instead of seeing it as a kind of personal call, like Joan of Arc hearing voices, it is trivialised: carers are just doing their job. For example, this was the justification of people who did not want to applaud them from their balcony: 'Do people applaud me when I go to work? They are paid for it'. In any salaried job, there may be more intense moments, justifying a request for a pay rise, just as the carers did (successfully). This does not mean that they should be applauded.

I. Sainsaulieu, *Care Staff Mobilisation in the Hospital*,
https://doi.org/10.1007/978-981-19-9354-1_4

That said, care work is not a trivial job. First of all, it is highly legitimate socially, like the work of firefighters, whether they are volunteers or paid employees. Rescuers are also popular, as can be seen during storms or floods, when ordinary workers and rescuers cooperate in urgent work. On 11 September 2001, all of America applauded the workers and firefighters who came to help. On a smaller scale, workers are in the foreground during storms, when they mobilise on the roofs of hospitals.

Healthcare probably makes everyone even more aware of their own vulnerability, because everyone has been in hospital and due to the ordinary confrontation of life and death. Just as one cannot reduce professional commitment to the presence of the patient, since it is based primarily on mastery of one's work perimeter and, therefore, on control of the patient, so one cannot forget the patient in care. By treating a person, there is a stake of compassion in the face of others, a reminder of one's own humanity, according to Levinas. There is an obvious ethical dimension to care. Moreover, the risk taken by healthcare workers was evident during the pandemic. We could and should applaud carers who took care of the common good, of human life endangered by the pandemic, including their own.

Contrary to what one might think, mobilisation in healthcare is not a natural state, inherent in a professional activity. Mobilising against the pandemic meant taking the risk of a significant state of fatigue. Already, in the face of the second wave, the carers we met at the end of 2020 were feeling the pinch. In the spring of 2021, absences due to illness increased, as in the case of the University Hospital Centre (CHU) where we carried out our survey, in eastern France. Not to mention the risk of contagion: in the same establishment, a thousand people contracted the virus, fortunately without any deaths attributable to it. In short, if we add the ordinary risks weighing on nurses (the high work rate, the lack of beds and staff), we can conclude that hospital staff already sorely tested by poor working conditions took on additional risks.

However, we will focus less on the 'halo' than on the particularities of ordinary care work. The latter conceals possibilities for building more egalitarian relationships in the workplace that are just as much, if not more, relevant to the fate of society. Thus, objectivist and subjectivist conceptions have emphasised the challenge of a more egalitarian society through this type of work carried out on others: the promises of the objective advent of the service society and the intersubjective struggle for a society of care.

## 4.1   Broken Promises of the Service Society

Using the evocative name of the 'service society', colleagues have described the promises of the rise of the tertiary sector (Delaunay & Gadrey, 1987). The core of this third sector being services, the authors saw the emergence of a 'service society', a society centred on the needs of users and no longer on individual profit. As the authors repeatedly denounced, the development of the service sector has been domesticated by capitalism, and the technological boom in communications has even given rise to the new pillars of capitalism, the GAFAM. Certainly, its players boast of giving access to greater freedom, but not for free: they get rich in a very traditional way by intensifying the work of engineers or unskilled workers, as in Amazon's parcel sorting centres.

As for the content of work, although trends have been affirmed in the formerly industrialised countries (a multi-century decline in the arduousness of work, qualification, growth of the service economy and feminisation of employment), the industrial service society remains polarised. In Germany, on the one hand there is an 'aristocracy' of expert managers with 'structural power', autonomous and competitive, and on the other hand regiments of unskilled workers experiencing domination, the 'service proletariat' (Nachtwey, 2020, p. 86). On the basis of an average stagnation of labour income, despite an increase in productivity, the wage gap is growing. Thirty million German wage earners ('the bottom 40% of German households') have seen their income stagnate or fall since the 1990s, and relative poverty affected 16% of the population in 2010 (Nachtwey, ibid.). In Germany, once a social democratic model, the increase in inequality is spectacular, even if it is held back by redistribution mechanisms. Precarity accounts for a growing share of new hires and, therefore, affects young people and unskilled work in particular.

Despite or because of these inequalities, it is important to know whether the service sector itself generates different struggles from the industrial sector (Sainsaulieu, 2017). In a sense, the service relationship at the heart of many service activities (care, teaching, trade, social work, etc.) can constitute a specific issue for mobilisation. Thus, in home help, the professional struggles of home helpers were supported in the neighbourhood where the employees usually worked (Avril, 2009). Similarly, the neighbourhood 'community' can be mobilised to support the employees of a retirement home (McAlevey, 2016). Professionals may denounce the loss of quality in their work and find an echo in the population, due to the concomitant deterioration in the service provided to the population. The meaning of the service relationship can also have an internal connotation within the service company. For example, unqualified employees in the retail sector were able to turn the internal family spirit against their company when the management changed its internal policy. Whereas the retention of employees through internal promotion compensated for a dull and low-paying job, the recruitment of external managers and the desire to increase margins changed the human resources policies of many retail companies, such as Walmart in the US, Carrefour in France or Migros in Switzerland. Internal promotion has given way to more external, more competitive recruitment. Employees in large-scale retailing then sometimes invoked this family spirit and turned it against the managers accused of deviating from it (Hocquelet, 2014).

### Micro-social or Macro-social Process?

On the other hand, workers' victories have depended here as elsewhere on strategy, especially trade union strategy. The unions are more or less aware of the transversal necessities of organising, defined as a quantitative and qualitative strategy that relies on the association of as many workers as possible with the collective decisions that concern them and on the emergence of new mediating leaders (McAlevey, 2016).

Regretting the excessive normativity of industrial relations, a subdiscipline whose research agenda is under the continuous influence of the authorities (Kelly, 1998, p. 23), John Kelly redefined its contours by drawing on the sociology of mobilisations. Claiming the hybridisation of the two sub-fields, he underlines the contributions of the latter. Thus, with the triptych 'organise-mobilise-seize opportunities', Tilly (quoted by Kelly, p. 25) proposes to investigate both the inclusive capacity of the organisational structure (e.g. its degree of centralisation), its capacity to mobilise resources and to group individuals together and to seize opportunities to maximise gains and minimise losses. In summary, collective action can take different forms depending on the balance achieved between interests, organisation, mobilisation and opportunities (Kelly, p. 26). In doing so, the focus is on 'transformational leaders' who bridge these components. Through discussion, reframing and ideology, simple elements (individuals, feelings of injustice, identities, interests) can be transformed by the mediation of these leaders into more elaborate elements (collectives, consciousness, commitments, strategies, collective action, demands).

At the same time, colleagues have emphasised the social context. They agree that 'the real degree of group organisation' varies widely according to the 'social process', defined as the degree of identification of members with their organisation and the 'degree of interaction, or density of social ties' (Kelly, 1998, p. 37). Whatever the quality of the leader, a sociological mystery thus remains, opening up the analysis of the daily activist practices of framing within 'micromobilisation contexts' (McAdam, quoted in conclusion), on which academic knowledge would remain 'astonishingly slight' (Kelly, p. 54).

However, it is rather towards macro-sociological factors that Kelly turns, illuminating the decline of trade unionism by the 'counter-mobilisation' of the 'capitalist state' and establishing a correlation between the ups and downs of worker protest and those of Kondratieff economic cycles ('long waves'). In particular, periods of transition between business cycles are associated with 'dramatic changes in indicators of industrial relations': union formation and development, strike activity, collective agreements, participatory management (p. 106).

Despite his homage to the 'social process', Kelly thus develops arguments that are more political and economic than properly sociological. In fact, the key political factors are fairly timeless or cyclical (militant activism, strike activity, counter-mobilisation or state repression), like economic cycles. However, unlike economic cycles, whose endogenous cause (the anarchy of the system or the invisible hand of the market) is well known, political factors can be understood as causes as well as consequences. Above all, if militant presence, state repression or strike activity play a certain role, are we to believe that they are in a perpetual cyclical renewal? We are left wondering about the history and analysis of the social transformations that accompany the evolution of a wage relationship. If the latter is part of the foundation of capitalist society, it does not escape a materialist history where the modalities of the social relation are redefined.

The author rightly refutes the metaphysical evolutionary reasoning of postmodernism and seems to be quick to point out the socio-economic phenomenon of the rise of the tertiary sector. Indeed, he is content to recall, rightly, that the latter is included in capitalist production. But on the one hand, if there is a disguised secondary sector (workers are referred to differently in the parent company and in the subsidiary depending on it), there is also an inflationary surge in occupations that do not depend on industry directly but on personal services (Nachtwey, 2020). In contrast, industry is growing enormously in other emerging countries of the South, whereas this was rare in the days of the colonial empires.

## A Sluggish Historical Driving Force

The service trades include a strong dualisation and pluralisation: while there is a strong contrast between skilled and unskilled trades, there is also a diversification of activities which prevents the new proletarians from being grouped into a social status of the precariat. We can compare them rather to the peasants' sack of potatoes, a Marxian metaphor to underline the contrast between the similarity of the peasants' living conditions and their inability to unite due to the lack of contacts between them. From this point of view, the large-scale industry at the time of the Industrial Revolution has not been replaced quantitatively and qualitatively by a new driving force of history in the countries of the North, even if it is developing in the South. Although the economic cycles remain, with their phases of growth and crisis, they are no longer based on an industrial revolution and are no longer forced into technological innovation by competition from the USSR. Profits are made within capitalist groups that have never been so global. The division of labour is international within them, while it has partly changed at the level of nations. A kind of 'internationalism' is manifested today in the renewed appetites of nation-states or politico-religious currents seeking to restore an imperial dimension. Thus, Russia, China and Turkey are threatening, and Africa is once again a battleground. An inter-imperial rivalry of unhappy memory has resurfaced between the two new antagonistic powers, China and the US.

In the social history of the French proletariat, colleagues have highlighted the forces of national integration. If the proletarians paid for it with two world wars, an integrative trend absorbed the 'nomadic' proletarians of the nineteenth century (Perrot, 1973) and separated them from the 'status employees' of the twentieth century, divided between social security, consumerism and downgrading (Castel, 1995; Nachtwey, 2020). It is not so much the sense of the collective that has been lost as the sense of revolution, the desire to change society. If anger still rumbles in the underprivileged working class, it does not affect all employees, especially those in large companies, and even less so in the long term. Immigrant proletarians have been integrated like their predecessors, even though injustice becomes more striking with the widening of inequalities. Thus the anger of the Yellow Vests in France did not concern employees of large companies, nor the young people of foreign origin grouped in the suburbs. The recent deaths in the suburbs of Marseille, Guadeloupe and Mayotte are largely the product of struggles between gangs for control of drug sales. A downward spiral involving strike action, de-unionisation and de-industrialisation has been going on for decades and is being seen on a global scale.

As for the content of consumer exchanges, it is not subversive. Individual and collective networks exist, and each of us has seen our planetary existence extended by dematerialising through social networks or communication technologies (including the latest, Zoom). But these networks do not necessarily broaden horizons; this depends largely on the actuality of social change. The intensification of networks otherwise largely reproduces the pre-existing social order. Their social elasticity is not phenomenal but is largely within diverse families, literally and figuratively, which reinforce internal links, even localism. The far right is the first to take advantage of narrow-mindedness, the taste for the 'people', the esoteric, and even the irrational and conspiracies that proliferate there. Connectivity does not necessarily lead to open-mindedness, social mixing and emancipation.

In this context, the promises of changing social relations in care work are of great interest.

## 4.2   CARE SOCIETY AND CARE WORK

As we have discussed elsewhere, the universalist conception of justice has not been entirely successful in convincing people that it offers guarantees for the claims of socially minority categories (Barozet, Sainsaulieu, Cortesero, & Mélo, 2022). The ethics of care aim to reconfigure the conception of justice in such a way as to include them, or at least to make it more difficult to ignore them. Indeed, care ethics express values that are often marginalised, such as caring or responsibility for others. One theorist of black feminism points out that the ethic of care corresponds in particular to the values of African-American communities—where the denigration of emotions and their separation from cognition are thought to be less. These values can be understood from 'an epistemology of connection' based on 'attention to the other' (Hill Collins, 2008). The project of a 'care society' thus encourages practices based on taking into account one's own vulnerability as well as that of others. This response cannot be based solely on the contribution of those who provide care but calls for a 'fairer redistribution of tasks and responsibilities' within a 'politics of care' (Paperman & Molinier, 2011).

Is gender, therefore, a vector of moralisation? According to Paperman and Molinier (2011), Carole Gilligan makes justice and care two rival voices, but present in each of us, the voice of care being, according to her, less quickly stifled in girls than in boys. The ethics of care, by explicitly opening up the perspective of a 'different moral voice', has created a new field of reflection, by placing the two moral voices in rivalry, or even on an equal footing: a morality centred on fairness, impartiality and autonomy, and valued by a tradition of thought that can be identified as masculine; and a morality formulated 'in a different voice', most often recognised in the experience of women, and based on the preservation and maintenance of human bonds. In identifying this difference, Carol Gilligan did not so much aim to introduce an essential difference as to highlight our assumptions about morality and the stifling of a voice in all of us (Paperman & Molinier, 2011). In her book (Gilligan, 2019) and in her interviews, Carol Gilligan clearly contrasts a patriarchy-dominated feminist ethic with a democratic feminist ethic. Indeed, care ethics are based on an analysis of the historical conditions that have fostered a division of moral labour, whereby caring activities have been socially and morally devalued. The historically documented assignment of women to the domestic sphere has reinforced the rejection of these activities and concerns from the public sphere. Conversely, the care society perspective calls for a reduction in working time for men, to recognise 'the reality of workers' multiple responsibilities for earning and caring by reducing the standard for full-time work and increasing vacation and leave time' (Glenn, 2000, p. 93).

American feminist thought was relayed in France with a time lag, but then caught up. Another French-speaking author, Christelle Avril (2018), has reported on the work of Joan Tronto (1993, published in French in 2009), but this time from a critical perspective aimed at distinguishing a normative approach from a heuristic one. For Avril, Joan Tronto defends a new social contract centred on the recognition of interpersonal relations of care (and dependence) to others, rather than on political rights in the classical sense of the term. This brings us back to the distinction between abstract masculine and concrete feminine morality mentioned above. On the moral and political level, the project makes visible the role played by 'certain categories that are more providers of care than others', such as women and immigrants, even though all individuals need care that they cannot provide for themselves. But the author wants to distinguish between a category of analysis and a normative category aiming to bring about a society based on the ethics of care. According to Joan Tronto (and Berenice Fisher), 'care is a generic activity that includes everything we do to maintain, perpetuate and repair our "world" so that we can live in it as well as possible. This world includes our bodies, ourselves and our environment, all of which we seek to link together in a complex, life-supporting network' (Tronto, 2009, p. 143).

The general nature of the definition allows it to be applied to all human activities but, in so doing, can give the impression of working 'every time' in the field of investigation, whereas 'a notion that applies to all human activities is not very, if at all, heuristic for an empirical sociologist' (Avril et al., 2010, p. 12). While the perspective of care opens up stimulating avenues of analysis for the sociology of service occupations, where women from working-class backgrounds are concentrated today, it is recommended that 'this term not be mobilised to describe and analyse work practices' (Avril, 2018). On the one hand, care makes visible or puts into perspective the emotions surrounding service work, while on the other hand it makes them invisible by indifferentiating them. The compassionate register in fact obeys very variable configurations, contrary to what care as a perspective might suggest. Thus, while care presupposes disinterestedness, carers may have an interest in this disinterestedness, like senior civil servants according to Bourdieu or militants according to Gaxie (Bourdieu, 2022; Gaxie, 2005): 'breaking the monotony', proving something to themselves. Care is in fact both a practice (caring for) and a disposition (caring about) according to Glenn (2000), distinct definitions that Hochschild and Tronto supposedly mixed up (Avril, 2018).

Care work may or may not reproduce domestic socialisation, female care. It is sometimes feminine and sometimes feminist. It is not predestined and is certainly often oriented by primary socialisation towards female sacrifice, but it is redefined during secondary socialisation (Ibos et al., 2019). 'The feminine ethic of care is indeed born in the soil of care, support and assistance activities that are assigned primarily to women as women, i.e. as they are socially defined through the maternal norm of devotion. However, this ethic does not mechanically reproduce the norms of self-sacrifice and dedication imposed on women' (Ibos et al., 2019, pp. 149–154). If the feminine ethic of care is embedded in the patriarchal ideology of self-sacrifice, the analysis of care work leads to a further step, by showing that through its works, the feminine ethic of care always exceeds and sometimes subverts the ideology of self-sacrifice. Thus, work accentuates the patriarchal heritage or, on the contrary, allows women to have a new relationship to qualification, a new way of socially constructing a female profession by purging it of any reference to 'natural' qualities and inscribing it in socially acquired skills, as nurses strongly claimed in 1989 (Kergoat, 1992).

But the balance seems to have tipped in the patriarchal direction. The work of nurses is apparently formally defined in the hospital by a strict technical division of labour. However, a close examination reveals a traditional function of a woman doing everything, in the role of the broom wagon in a cycling race. So, women nurses or care assistants, like women in the social sector, are morally responsible for doing 'what remains to be done' (Avril & Ramos Vacca, 2020). They are the custodians of the dirty work mentioned by Hugues and get their hands dirty for others. At the bottom of the moral division of labour, they carry out the tasks that hamper the institution or defend its failings, through increased surveillance or lies, in particular by covering up the failings of doctors: 'he's not here because he's been held up in a meeting' (Avril & Ramos Vacca, 2020). Worse, they have to invent from scratch operation reports that surgeons did not take the time to make.

More broadly, care work currently appears to be more of a social constraint than a means of emancipation for women. Thus, care work in the US appears to be at the intersection of two interconnected strands: unpaid domestic care and slavery, or other forms of forced labour (Glenn, 2000). The result of this pattern is a devaluation of care work and the exclusion of unpaid and paid care workers from basic rights such as the minimum wage, pension benefits and workers' compensation. A whole conception of gender, family, race and citizenship has shaped the development of care work and social policy, leading in particular to immigrant women and women of colour doing a disproportionate share of care work (Glenn, 2000). In the same vein, Maud Simonet denounces the exploitation of those who care for people in a voluntary capacity. The denial of the work done makes it all the easier for others to appropriate it. In a field study on unpaid public work (*gratuitisation*), using the example of the upkeep of public spaces in the US and France, the author highlights the way in which local councils have managed to cope with budgetary restrictions by mobilising two categories of the population whose work could be carried out outside of the traditional representations of work: volunteers and recipients of social assistance programmes (Simonet, 2018).

Elsa Dorlin even inverts the value of care, by questioning what she calls negative or dirty care (Dorlin, 2017). According to essentialist visions, women are deemed attentive and considerate, which explains their readiness to look after others and, therefore, to work in the caring professions. Negative care, Elsa Dorlin tells us, is also the attention paid to others, but not in order to take care of them: it is a question of escaping harassment, rape, and the daily violence exercised by men on women. It is the attention of the prey to the predator. In this relationship, as in all relationships of domination, it is the object (the hunter) that dominates the subject (the prey insofar as it exercises its cognitive capacities), because it is its point of view that defines the real, a real that some authors, quoted in a footnote by Elsa Dorlin, remind us that English and Spanish etymology relate to 'expressions that refer to "royal" or that are relative to the king'. What is real is what is visible to the king. The other effect of this negative care concerns the 'king-object'. It has already been designated by the concept of agnotology, the study of the production of ignorance. Unlike prey, which must know as much as possible about their predators in order to hope to escape them, predators have no need to know more about their prey. This is in line with the idea that listening carries political values, linked to care and emancipation, as a social behaviour that respects people and carries 'resistance to the patriarchal framework' (Gilligan, 2009).

## 4.3    Hesitant Alternative Care Practices

The pressures in terms of finances and capacity-facing health systems are prompting the search for new strategies to provide effective and quality services. Thus, 'bricolage' appears to be a central notion in describing care practices, just as forging invisible links seems to be inherent in care-framing practices (Bourret, 2006).

The proponents of new technologies promised to revolutionise care, just as they promised to change the world (Sainsaulieu & Saint-Martin, 2019). A recent book has taken a closer look at the relationship between care and technology, seeking to rethink their relations. Technology is shifting, surprising and adaptable, integrable in changing care practices. In the latter, all 'things' are (and must be) constantly changing, while knowledge is also fluid: rather than a set of general rules, knowledge relevant to care practices is adaptable and must be adapted to both technologies and bodies, to people and the daily lives involved (Mol et al., 2010). This mutual adaptation is, therefore, not about a revolution in care.

More extensive experiments have taken place on some occasions (more on this below). In the field of HIV, practices have kept lasting traces of the 'AIDS revolution', as former infectious disease nurses say (Sainsaulieu, 2012). Similarly, in three New York City clinics specialising in HIV care, colleagues have shown how HIV care is the result of a daily co-production between professionals and patients (Baim Lance et al., 2018). An ethnographic approach based on 'health practices' guided the exploration of patients' activities, their effects on clinical processes and the conditions surrounding their performance. The article shows how co-production is forged by building relationships within the clinic, and with patients, within a wider human community. These dynamics reveal how patients' bodily and temporal understandings are integrated and shape the co-produced services.

However, this innovative constraint has real limitations. In this post-Covid period, there are reports of many nurses resigning in search of less trying situations than those they experienced in the public hospital, whether French, Swiss or, as here, Canadian: 'In the public sector, we drag out the 16-hour shifts, it's the quality of life that suffers, family life, the children we can't pick up from daycare because we're held back at work with compulsory overtime', says a nurse interviewed by a Canadian online newspaper (*Le journal du Québec*, 26 July 2021, Vague de démission infirmière, Jean Houle).

In fact, ethical innovation still seems to be an avant-garde practice, as the limits seem to be so important.

First, there are limits specific to the medical profession. Traditionally, doctors have rejected the contributions of the nursing sciences. Recent developments show that the boundary remains rigid. Nurses are exploring the universe of possibilities, broadening their scope of action and engaging in what can be conceptualised as an ethic of healing, implying a nursing discipline that implements practices that lead to healing. However, this approach is rejected by the medical profession at all levels (Ernst, 2020). Similarly, new technologies can increase the skills and responsibilities of nurses, as in the example of telecare via screen-mediated conferences. In telecare, greater accountability, discretion and responsibility are imposed on the nurse, but she also has less access to the clinical decision-making capabilities of physicians. The nurse is thus given greater responsibility while becoming more dependent on the physician (Nickelsen & Niels, 2019).

Doctors also tend to ignore the contribution of their subordinates, the locums, who are perceived as inferior to permanently employed doctors in terms of quality, skill and safety. Locums are often stigmatised, marginalised and even excluded (Ferguson et al., 2020).

Together, caregivers may also exclude non-caregivers. Thus, healthcare systems focus primarily on 'curing disease' and ignore the essential work of the professions at the bottom, including community support workers, who are truly 'marginal and invisible care providers' (Parsons, 2021). The hospital-outside-the-walls intervention teams also have difficulty in existing and gaining recognition from the hospital world (Sainsaulieu & Vega, 2014). Even intra-hospital mobile teams have difficulty gaining acceptance in care services, as in the example of geriatric and palliative care mobile teams, made up of geriatric doctors and paramedics who have difficulty asserting their expertise in the specialised care services of hospitals in northern France (Castra & Sainsaulieu, 2020).

A colleague has shown the manifestation and consequences of the formal boundaries of hospital departments (Nugus, 2019). Noting the same dramatic compartmentalisation, he questions the prevalence of stable order over the famous notion of negotiated order in hospitals (Strauss, 1992). Compared to inpatient hospital services, emergency departments have limited legitimacy to claim organ-specific knowledge, especially for transferring patients from the emergency department. The manifestation of hierarchies of specialised knowledge in organisational structures penalises older and chronically ill patients, highlighting the effects of stable organisational orders.

Finally, the public relations aspect is not much better. Hospitals in Scotland are struggling to make changes or closures clear to the public because of a failure to rethink mechanisms for public involvement by prioritising processes of dialogue. Colleagues sometimes see these public relations as a trace of class contempt: for example, new manifestations of stigma and blame are emerging in austerity Britain. Increasing working-class blame is aided and abetted by the mainstream media for poor health and lifestyle 'choices' and 'behaviour'. Those who previously relied on safety nets such as sickness and disability benefits are increasingly rejected by the state and accused of being 'slackers' or 'fraudsters' (Scambler, 2018). Similarly, in France, the public debate is increasingly taken up with the issue of fraud by recipients of social benefits (Dubois & Lieutaud, 2020).

In this way, ethics is presented as doubly impoverished: in the social sense of taking into consideration fractured situations (Scambler, 2018) and in the professional sense of non-medical, or even non-paramedical skills in care. If institutional and professional arrangements offer no alternative, should the transgression of norms not come from the mobilisation of the carers themselves?

## BIBLIOGRAPHY

Avril, C. (2009). Une mobilisation collective dans l'aide à domicile à la lumière des pratiques et des relations de travail. *Politix, 86*, 97–118.

Avril, C. (2018). 15—Sous le *care*, le travail des femmes de milieux populaires. Pour une critique empirique d'une notion à succès. In M. Maruani (Ed.), *Je travaille, donc je suis. Perspectives féministes* (pp. 205–216). La Découverte.

Avril, C., Cartier, M., & Serre, D. (2010). *Enquêter sur le travail: Concepts, méthodes, récits.* Paris: La Découverte.

Avril, C., & Ramos Vacca, I. (2020). Se salir les mains pour les autres. Métiers de femme et division morale du travail. *Travail, genre et sociétés, 43*, 85–102.

Baim-Lance, A., Tietz, D., Lever, H., Swart, M., & Agins, B. (2018). Everyday and Unavoidable Coproduction: Exploring Patient Participation in the Delivery of Healthcare Services. *Sociology, Health and Illness, 41*(1), 128–142. https://doi.org/10.1111/1467-9566.12801

Barozet, E., Sainsaulieu, I., Cortesero, R., & Mélo, D. (2022). *Where Has Social Justice Gone? From Equality to Experimentation.* Palgrave Macmillan.

Bourdieu, P. (2022). *L'intérêt au désintéressement. Cours au collège de France, 1987–1988.* Seuil.

Bourret, P. (2006). *Les cadres de santé à l'hôpital. Un travail de lien invisible.* Ed. Seli Arsan.

Castel, R. (1995). *Les métamorphoses de la question sociale* (p. 490). Une chronique du salariat. Fayard.

Castra, M., & Sainsaulieu, I. (2020). Intervenir sur un autre territoire professionnel. Equipes mobiles et services sédentaires à l'hôpital. *Sciences sociales et santé, 38*(4), 47–74.

Delaunay, J.-C., & Gadrey, J. (1987). *Les enjeux de la société de service.* Presses de Science Po.

Dorlin, E. (2017). *Se défendre. Une philosophie de la violence.* Zones éditions.

Dubois, V., & Lieutaud, M. (2020). La 'fraude sociale' en questions. La naturalisation d'une thématique politique au prisme des questions à l'assemblée nationale (1986–2017). *Revue française de science politique, 70*(3–4), 341–371.

Ernst, J. (2020). Professional Boundary Struggles in the Context of Healthcare Change: The Relational and Symbolic Constitution of Nursing Ethos in the Space of Possible Professionalisation. *Sociology, Health and Illness, 42*(7), 1727–1741. https://doi.org/10.1111/1467-9566.13161

Ferguson, J., Tazzyman, A., Walshe, K., Bryce, M., Boyd, A., Archer, J., Price, T., & Tredinnick-Rowe, J. (2020). 'You're just a locum': Professional Identity and

Temporary Workers in the Medical Profession. *Sociology, Health and Illness,* *43*(1), 149–166. https://doi.org/10.1111/1467-9566.13210

Gaxie, D. (2005). Rétributions du militantisme et paradoxes de l'action collective. *Swiss Political Science Review, 11*(1), 157–188.

Gilligan, C. (2009). Le care, éthique féminine ou éthique féministe? *Multitudes, 37–38*(2–3), 76–78.

Gilligan, C. (2019). *Une voix différente. La morale a-t-elle un sexe?* Champs-Essais.

Glenn, E. N. (2000). Creating a Caring Society. *Contemporary Sociology, 29*, 84–94.

Hill Collins, P. (2008). La construction sociale de la pensée féministe Noire. In E. Dorlin (Dir.), *Black Feminism, Anthologie du féminisme africain-américain, 1975–2000* (pp. 135–175). L'Harmattan.

Hocquelet, M. (2014). Les passés composés de la grande distribution: De l'appropriation managériale au support des contestations salariales. *Sociologies pratiques, 29*, 63–72.

Ibos, C., Damamme, A., Molinier, P., & Paperman, P. (2019). Le *care* justifie le sacrifice des femmes. Dans: Ibos, Damamme, Molinier, & Paperman (Dir.), *Vers une société du care. Une politique de l'attention.* Le Cavalier Bleu.

Kelly, J. (1998). *Rethinking Industrial Relations. Mobilization, Collectivism and Long Waves.* Routledge.

Kergoat, D. (1992). *Les infirmières et leur coordination, 1988–1989* (p. 192). Editions Lamarre.

McAlevey, J. (2016). *No Shortcuts: Organizing for Power in the New Gilded Age.* Oxford University Press.

Moll, A., Moser, I., & Pols, J. (2010). *Care in Practice: On Tinkering in Clinics, Homes and Farms.* Transcript Verlag. https://doi.org/10.14361/transcript.9783839414477

Nachtwey, O. (2020). *La société du déclassement. La contestation à l'ère de la modernité régressive.* Editions de la Maison des Sciences de l'Homme.

Nickelsen, M., & Niels, C. (2019). The Infrastructure of Telecare: Implications for Nursing Tasks and the Nurse-Doctor Relationship. *Sociology, Health and Illness, 41*(1), 67–80.

Nugus, P. (2019). Re-structuring the Negotiated Order of the Hospital. *Sociology, Health and Illness, 41*(2), 378–394. https://doi.org/10.1111/1467-9566.12838

Paperman, P., & Molinier, P. (2011). L'éthique du care comme pensée de l'égalité. *Travail, genre et sociétés, 2011/2*, n° 26, 89–193.

Parsons, S. (2021). Support Workers and the Health Professions in International Perspective. *The Invisible Providers of Health Care, Mike Saks, Bristol: Policy Press, Sociology, Health and Illness, 43*(7), 1720–1721. https://doi.org/10.1111/1467-9566.13303

Perrot, M. (1973). *Les Ouvriers en grève. France 1871–1890.* Mouton.

Sainsaulieu, I. (2012). Collective Mobilisation in Hospitals: Confrontational or Consensual? *Revue française de sociologie (English)*, 53(3), 316–346.

Sainsaulieu, I. (2017). *Conflits et résistances au travail* (p. 150). SciencesPo Les Presses, coll. "Contester".

Sainsaulieu, I., & Vega, A. (2014). Introduction. *Les Sciences de l'éducation—Pour l'Ère nouvelle, 47*(3), 7–11.

Sainsaulieu, I., & Saint-Martin, A. (Eds.). (2019). *L'innovation en eaux troubles. Sciences, techniques, idéologies* (p. 329). Editions du Croquant.

Scambler, G. (2018). *Sociology, Health, and the Fractured Society: A Critical Realist Account* (p. 208). Routledge.

Simonet, M. (2018). *Travail gratuit, la nouvelle exploitation*. Editions Textuel.

Strauss, A. (1992). *La trame de la negotiation*. L'Harmattan.

Tronto, J. (2009). *Un monde vulnérable, pour une politique du care* (*Moral Boundaries: A Political Argument for an Ethic of Care*, 1993). La Découverte.

# CHAPTER 5

# Spontaneous Protest

**Abstract** The opposition between bureaucracy and mobilisation takes a more concrete turn here by opposing two social types on the occasion of an emergency strike: *homo mobilis* versus *homo immobilis*. We can see how the strikers ingeniously created an interconnection network of hospital emergencies, while the network pre-established by the unions was not mobilised. The need to organise autonomously is felt because of the many professional frustrations of the carers and the wait-and-see attitude of the official organisations. We also question the brakes on the protest mobilisation of carers, such as the assignment of strikers within the framework of continuity of care, to ask ourselves whether self censorship due to guilt is not stronger than legal assignment in curbing recourse to strike action.

**Keywords** Spontaneity • Nursing • Self-organisation • Emergency room strike

The 'malaise of carers' (Sainsaulieu, 2003) has been an omnipresent reality in hospitals since the 1980s. The long-term policy of reducing salary costs in public hospitals affects all non-medical staff. As a result, professionals and managers suffer from not doing the job that corresponds to their professional ideal, the one for which they were trained and prepared, sometimes for a long period.

I. Sainsaulieu, *Care Staff Mobilisation in the Hospital*, https://doi.org/10.1007/978-981-19-9354-1_5

At the same time, it is precisely this ideal that allows them to endure the ordeal. The expression of job dissatisfaction in conflictual terms is therefore not a priori obvious, as we have seen. Caregivers are capable of mobilising themselves in their work with collective and egalitarian logics without engaging in protest. Nevertheless, the deterioration of their working conditions has also led them to demand better material conditions.

It is this ambivalence between consensus and contestation that we will deal with in this chapter, showing how the incomplete construction of the nursing profession weighs on consensual mobilisation, on the one hand, and how the organisational and institutional hierarchy determines the modalities for moving to contestation, on the other.

## 5.1   Nursing, a Thwarted Profession

In France, the question of nurses' professional identity is a recurrent one. While in other countries nurses may have achieved genuine academic and hospital positions, the social and hierarchical position of nurses remains far below that of doctors. Although nurses are the dominant paramedical body in hospitals, they are not alone. Nurses' aides make up the other paramedical care component. However, while nurses have had and continue to have a problem with their professional identity, care assistants have less corporate ambition. Coming from working-class backgrounds to a greater extent than nurses (Sainsaulieu, 2014), nurses' aides have stronger ties with the working class or hospital employees and with trade unions, on the one hand, and with patients and their families, on the other. They tend to 'turn the stigma' of being low-ranking employees on its head and emphasise their attachment to the patient's well-being (Arborio, 2009).

On the contrary, since its emergence at the end of the nineteenth century, the nursing professional group has been working for better social, salary, symbolic and scientific 'recognition' by demanding, in particular, longer training, a higher level diploma, a wider range of authorised acts, the development of the nursing sciences, the integration of research into their training and missions, better pay, autonomy in relation to medical power and the reinforcement of their political representation with the authorities, in the form of associations, trade unions and professional associations.

What quest is of greater interest to professionals than that of their professionalisation, this process of recognition, autonomy of categories of workers and their stabilisation and legitimisation as professional groups (Demazière, 2009)? This quest can be summed up as a desire to conquer one's own territory, 'the issues of mastery, control and configuration of work [being] more or less universal among all professional groups' (Demazière, 2009). However, these are not necessarily isolated struggles. The struggle to define the boundaries of the professions involves not only segments of the professions but also their historically determined allies in the state, among private or even commercial players, or civic actors (associations, ethnic groups). Each social world (professional, political, economic, associative, cultural, etc.) constitutes a particular ecology, including a particular place, players and links. Struggles bring certain segments into conflict with those of other ecologies, thus forming 'linked ecologies', as in the case of doctors in New York State (Abbott, 2003). Intra- or interprofessional struggles are, therefore, political because of the alliances with other players, in particular, state players.

French nurses have partially entered into such a process of professional socialisation. Following numerous struggles and bitter discussions with interlocutors who were not very permeable or even hostile, and also because of the stimulating foreign models cited to underline 'French backwardness' (North America, the UK, Australia, etc.), and with the support of some doctors, state regulation was put in place. Laws and decrees have officially ratified developments that are considered more or less positive, if not by nurses then at least by their spokespersons.

We can mention the bachelor's degree for nurses with a state diploma (IDE) introduced in 2009, the re-engineering of nursing specialities with the creation of a master's degree for IADEs (state-qualified anaesthetist nurses) or a master's degree currently under discussion for nurses with childcare responsibilities (Divay & Vega, 2022). Operating theatre nurses (IBODE) can move on to become health managers after four years of practice or become advanced practice nurses, while health managers are increasingly obtaining a master's degree through agreements between their training institutes (IFCS) and universities, particularly in management sciences. Finally, new master's degrees have recently appeared: for clinical nurse specialists (ISC) and above all for advanced practice nurses (IPA) in 2018, who can also claim specific positions that are more or less institutionalised: so-called referent nurses, coordinators, experts and more. In connection with this, section 92 in nursing sciences was created at the National Council of Universities, signifying the opening up of an academic nursing career.

Despite these recent developments, the nursing career remains under-resourced and does not result in an improvement in the quality of care provided in hospitals, on the contrary (Gheorghui & Vega, 2019). On the one hand, the less prestigious specialties (such as geriatrics or general med-icine) are forgotten or have even been invaded, such as the specialised nursing course in psychiatry, which was abolished in 1992 and integrated into the general nursing curriculum. On the other hand, newly qualified nurses have very little extra pay and time for clinical research. In practice, they are mainly used to manage medical shortages on the cheap, as doctors can save medical time by offloading work to auxiliaries who are more qual-ified than the 'basic nurse' while keeping control over their knowledge. So, all master's degrees in nursing are taught in medical school, while their new responsibilities in practice are duly framed by medical care protocols, sometimes generating strong bitterness linked to nursing-role expecta-tions, notably regarding the improvement of the quality of care. Indeed, managers are less and less available for their teams, and see families and patients less and less often, but spend more time codifying practices or managing schedules, following a number of untimely work stoppages by nurses. Young nurses in training are less supported and so feel less involved in the establishment's projects. It is said in the departments that the man-ager must 'mourn the death of the nursing profession' (Divay & Vega, 2022). As for the nursing directors at the top of the paramedical pyramid, this is a body whose numbers are falling year after year due to a lack of succession. The position is losing its attractiveness and is considered to be difficult and poorly paid when compared to other positions in hospital management (Divay & Girard, 2019).

Last but not least, the mass of hospital nurses is forgotten. The empha-sis placed on access to master's degrees by the group's national representa-tives (associations, National Order of Nurses, unions, nurses in advisory positions at the Ministry, etc.) concerns only a minority. In all, less than 10% of nurses are specialised, even though their proportion has increased by an annual average of 0.14% since 2000 (Divay, 2013). According to the Drees figures (https://drees.shinyapps.io/demographie-ps/), in 2021 there were 764,000 qualified nurses in France, of whom almost 500,000 were employed in hospitals, that is, more than two-thirds. In comparison, of the 230,000 doctors, only one-third are hospital doctors (72,000). The public authorities only grant occasional bonuses to nurses, as during the pandemic.

Seeking the allegiance of the public authorities, the representatives of the nursing profession contribute above all to social peace: in exchange for a few advances (the financial cost of which is under control), they accept worse working conditions, as a trauma nurse clinician pointed out: 'We work just-in-time with a view to optimising the workforce (…) It is a question of optimising care, speeding up re-education, bringing forward the return home, and eliminating downtime' (Divay & Vega, 2022). On the contrary, in the absence of organised resistance, the entire nursing profession is being swept along on a wave of managerial rationalisation, undermining nurses' professional identity by degrading their working conditions. Thus, a recent IPA graduate in a psychiatric hospital testifies that she sees 'no enhancement of working conditions, nor any militancy regarding the values of the public institution and accessibility to care for the most disadvantaged, nor any cross-disciplinary approach offered to staff who wish for it, for the sake of an artificial consideration of the qualities and quantity of the work provided' (Divay & Vega, 2022).

As a result of these developments, the theme of the 'privatisation' of the public hospital has become part of public consciousness and debate. Certain activities have indeed been privatised (cleaning, hotel services, laundry, ambulances, etc.), while private clinics manage part of the profitable hospital care, particularly surgery. But the state is forced to keep the least profitable activities, which consist mainly in caring for the most seriously ill patients. To compensate for this, it is trying to reduce salary costs by drawing on the managerial recipes of the private sector (Pierru, 2022). Contractual hiring has become widespread, instead of recruitment through competitive examinations.

But the lack of nurses makes it difficult to abolish their state-employee status. Faced with deteriorating working conditions, the best nurses are leaving to work elsewhere (private clinics, schools, etc.). The state is faced with a contradiction: making hospital work attractive, while at the same time reducing its costs, that is, the non-medical wage bill, with doctors having more means to defend themselves. It is not impossible that the state is counting on the general deterioration of working conditions for the working classes as a springboard to guarantee employment in hospitals, by lowering the levels of professionalism and driving out the middle classes. In his programme for re-election in April 2022, President Macron was not planning to hire new state employees, nor to stop the closure of beds, but to allow the monetisation of accumulated leave, to pay overtime, to raise the retirement age and to decrease unemployment benefits. Let's get to work!

## 5.2    SELF-ORGANISATION AND UNIONISM

As in the case of employees in large cultural stores, nurses experience a gap between the tasks they are given and their qualifications, which leads to great frustration. In the cultural sector, 'a feeling of routine, repetition of "robotic" tasks, limited initiative, low pay, no promotion prospects, surveillance and contempt from management, who tell them that they are only good for putting books on the shelves' all combine to feed their bitterness. Professional frustration is part of the pattern of relative frustration, fuelled by the observation that 'it is often not the most deprived [...] who revolt and engage in collective action' (Corcuff, 2009). The increase in qualifications and the rise in the reflexivity of the actors can lead to a strong self-commitment that raises the level of expectations, without them being paid back in the eyes of the players. This logic of professionalisation follows the rise in the average level of qualification of employees. Similarly, the manipulation of subjectivity by the new work organisations leads to disappointment, frustration and resistance (Linhart, 2015).

Does this professional frustration fuel union involvement? Sociologists differ about the role of unions in social movements. For some, the new social movements are the successors to the organised labour movement, due to the rise of a new society. For others, since the proletariat continues to exist, in the context of deteriorating working conditions, trade unionism remains relevant. It is still able to fight, especially in the service sector, where trade unionism has been revitalised in Germany (Verdi), France (Sud) and the US (SEIU).

Thus, in the example of nursing homes in Pennsylvania, at the heart of the 'rust belt', the battles waged show unions' renewed capacity to fight against large companies, through long-term campaigns. The author nevertheless recognises that the length of the struggle and the meagre results contrast with the lightning campaign of the CIO constitution in the 1930s. In Germany, the Verdi trade union only managed to wrest an unsatisfactory compromise from Deutsche Telekom in 2007 after six weeks of strike action: 50,000 employees were finally outsourced to the T-service subsidiary with a pay cut of 6.5%, instead of 9% and no redundancies for five years.

But the question that interests us here concerns the assimilation between trade unionism and the wage movement. In view of the unsatisfactory results of trade unionism, it is tempting for spontaneous movements of employee self-organisation to take over, as we saw during the well-known Yellow Vests movement (Sainsaulieu, 2020). As a result of developments in the history of the labour movement, democracy and the social state, trade unions have sharpened their dual nature. On the one hand, they play the role of a labour advocate. If employees have a problem with their management, they can get help from a trade union to defend their individual rights. On the other hand, this is not the case for the essential function found in the etymology of the term 'trade union': acting together. On the collective level, things have become more complex, with unions defending their place in the interface with the public authorities as much as, if not more than, engaging in collective action with workers.

In any case, discrepancies are perceptible between the union agenda and that of the workers: their calls for collective action do not always match the motivations of the work collective. They can be in the forefront, calling unexpected strikes, or lagging behind, taking a back seat when the workers want to mobilise. These discrepancies have been shown on several occasions by historians during major social movements, in France as well as in the US (Vigna, 2021; Fantasia & Voss, 2003).

They are a classic feature in the history of Marxism. Marx considered that trade unionism served to organise the workers' movement in its dual task of defending immediate interests and emancipating the proletariat (AIT, second congress, 1866, Geneva). This double task was expressed in the Amiens Charter, a fundamental orientation text of trade unionism adopted in 1906 at the CGT congress. Lenin later saw that trade unionism was content with immediate interests, leaving the revolutionary party with the task of dealing with general interests. For all that, he did not spare his criticisms of the Bolshevik Party, which was considered too timid in the face of the revolutionary audacity of the masses after the first revolution of February 1917. Trotsky extended this criticism, even calling for the creation of a new party beyond Stalinism.

On the anarchist side in the same period, the Industrial Workers of the World in the US notably challenged the classic syndicalism of the American Federation of Labour, accused of limiting itself to the conservative defence of a professional workers' aristocracy. They called for an industrial unionism dedicated to all workers (One Big Union) oriented towards a revolutionary overthrow of the bosses' class, capitalism and wage labour. They quickly divided between supporters of partisan political action (like Daniel De Léon) and partisans of direct action (like Big Bill Haywood), who were in the majority.

But, unlike in France, where revolutionary criticism persisted throughout the twentieth century as a legitimate model, including among renowned intellectuals, it seemed largely assimilated in the US. In any case, the constitution of the sociology of social movements was being renewed on the basis of the struggles for civil rights and feminism. The aspiration to empowerment and mobilisation, whether or not linked to electoral outlets, seemed to be connected to the democratic vitality of the community rather than to a revolutionary critique of institutions. In France, precursors such as Francois Chazel and Alain Touraine also closely linked democratisation and social movements, while a critique of wage work inspiring the sociology of work was maintained.

There is no doubt that May 1968 revitalised the critique of wage labour in France and even more so in Italy. In the post-1960s context, organising a social movement was not the prerogative of the unions which, in law, could just as well declare themselves to be the sole legitimate representatives of striking employees as consider themselves to be participants on the same basis as the others and let the employees themselves choose who should lead their movement. The right to strike is not entirely based on trade union rights: if the trade unions are the only ones legitimately permitted to give notice of a strike, which is a legal requirement in the public sector, the employee does not have to be a trade union member to make use of his or her right to strike a constitutional right since 1946.

In other words, alongside official-elected representatives in the bodies, there can be a self-organisation entirely designed ad hoc for the occasion. This is another democratic mechanism, that of direct democracy, which has a self-organisation to deal with a problem, in the same way as there are, in representative democracy, committees appointed by bodies to deal with a particular subject. The mechanism of direct democracy allows all those who want to do so to be fully involved in the action and to control it themselves. This is legitimised by the sacrifice made in strike action, with its own risks, making it legitimate and necessary for participants to have a say.

Many collective groupings were set up on these occasions, sometimes called strike committees, sometimes coordinations, sometimes transversal committees (inter-emergency, intensive care), on a local or national level, and most often reporting to a larger body (a general assembly of the personnel of the site or sites concerned). Only the strikers have the right to vote on the orientations and the right to elect their representatives within the committee created for the action.

Of course, employees are not equal when it comes to speaking in public, and permanent or professional activists have an advantage in imposing themselves as leaders. These assemblies are, therefore, also an arena where competition between experienced activists is played out. On the one hand, this democratic control can guarantee that the elected strike leaders take their instructions from the general assembly and not from a partisan or trade union apparatus outside the collective action; on the other hand, the wider and deeper the movement, the more it gives the opportunity to new entrants to play a role in the collective movement. These incoming leaders are then said to be 'revealed' in the movement—and they may disappear with it from the public scene or exercise their new sense of responsibility elsewhere.

If these principles of democratic life have been experienced in all professional sectors, they have been revitalised particularly in the care sector in recent years, from the nursing coordination in 1988–1989 to more recent collective movements, including the inter-emergency committee set up two years ago, which we will now examine.

## 5.3    A Self-Organised Movement in the Emergency Room

The emergency movement and the Inter-Emergency Collective (CIU) revived the nurses' coordination form of the 1988 movement. Once again, women affirmed their capacity to constitute themselves as 'social subjects', to put forward the relational side of care, in an inseparable relationship between content and self-managed form, even though the CIU demanded not only improvements in the nursing profession (by raising salaries and giving tenure to precarious workers) but also a halt to bed closures. This structure, which was born out of the emergency room movement, is typical of the self-organised structures that sometimes flourish during wage struggles in order to overcome or push back the limits of trade unionism (Gourgues, 2017; Sainsaulieu, 2020), by moving away from a trade union form that is 'too rigid'.

The CIU that we are going to examine was followed by other comparable initiatives, which we cite to better identify the limits of the spontaneous phenomenon. In the spring of 2021, while healthcare workers were facing the third wave of the pandemic, a call for a strike was issued for 11 May. Discontent was mounting: while healthcare workers had seen their working conditions slowly deteriorate for at least three decades (1990–2020), the pandemic had accelerated the process rather than halting it. Work flexibility had increased, with precarious staff representing a quarter of the workforce. The pandemic continued to depopulate other services, especially operating theatres, to support intensive care services. An intensive care movement called for strike action on 11 May 2021. It brought together intensive care workers in 105 cities. They called for the reinforcement of intensive care services by establishing a nurse/patient ratio, the creation of beds and permanent posts, a specific diploma and remuneration for intensive care staff. In Nice, 150 nursing staff staged a walkout in front of the hospital on 11 May, and everywhere in France the same slogan was displayed on hospital walls: 'Save your ICU, one day it will save you!'

### Summoning Strikers: Censorship or Self-Censorship?[1]

It is rare for paramedical staff in emergency services to go on strike (Ridel & Sainsaulieu, 2021). Striking care staff are assigned to their posts, sometimes well in advance, to maintain a minimum number of staff and ensure continuity of service. But there are many social aspects that modulate this ban.

Firstly, an emergency service is 'permanently understaffed', due to a lack of personnel. Organising a strike movement requires time, meetings and coordination between the care workers. However, high turnover prevents the establishment of a lasting professional sociability, as one carer testifies in a book written by a leader of the inter-emergency collective.

> We no longer build staff loyalty through contracts or tenure, and even less through salary. It's also a way for management to prevent staff from mobilising, because the longer you stay in the department, the better you know it, the closer the teams are and the more you are able to identify dysfunctions and demand changes. (Bleuenn, care assistant, in Huon, 2020, p. 234)

Secondly, strikes in emergency departments are invisible. They are generally short, localised, with changing causes: relocation, reorganisation, violence and so on. This fragmentation is accompanied by a lack of

---

[1] Acknowledgement: this passage (47–49) is derived from an article published in *Espace et Société*, ©Éditions Érès, Ridel Déborah, Sainsaulieu Ivan, 2021, 'Démobiliser les soignantes? Logiques spatiales, organisationnelles et institutionnelles à l'hôpital', 2-183, pp. 51–66.

coordination between the different departments. It is also accompanied by the social timidity of paramedical staff, who are less culturally and socially close to journalists than doctors. During the emergency room movement in 2018, the separation between doctors and paramedics persisted:

> While the conflict was led by paramedics for the first eight months, [the health minister] always addressed the doctors, accentuating the feeling of social injustice and class struggle. (Huon, 2020, p. 210)

Thus, the use of strike action is a socially differentiated practice—doctors and managers resort more easily to strike action—contrary to the law, which is egalitarian in principle. Moreover, the interpretation of this obligation remains individual, related to previous experiences and opinions.

Legal responsibility is also socially differentiated. The responsibility for what happens to patients lies primarily with hospital management. Moreover, it sometimes takes the initiative itself to close an emergency department and refer the public to another facility.

So, assigning patients to a hospital is above all a professional taboo that allows it to establish its legitimacy. For carers, it is morally difficult to consider abandoning patients. The self-blame of the staff is also pointed out by those who learn to protest through the strike.

That said, subordinate positions mean imposed work: assignment and sanctions threaten the humble first of all. In addition to self-censorship, there is the fear of repression through disciplinary action.

> Reprisals are real: measures such as reprimands, delays in tenure, moral harassment, the withdrawal of bonuses, etc. have been used frequently in recent months. (Huon, 2020, p. 311)

Pressure is a well-known register, ranging from summoning a striking nurse to explain herself to blackmail for tenure.

> During the strike, a colleague came to demonstrate at the hospital, the manager took a screenshot when she saw her on television. She sent it to her management, who summoned her. As she is a contract worker, the girl was dissuaded from continuing to follow the movement if she wanted to be hired on a permanent basis. (Claire, nurse, ibid., pp. 227–228)

*Mobilis Versus Immobilis: Two (Sub)species of Homo?*

However, hierarchical social relations are not the only obstacle to health-care workers' protests. They must also confront their unfaithful ally, the trade union apparatus.

An interview was posted online about the emergency room movement in 2019. It was conducted by the sociologist Pierre-André Juven with Hugo Huon, a nurse and president of the CIU, and Candice Lafarge, an orderly and spokesperson for the CIU. It shows us the gap between the movement and the unions, beyond the unionisation of certain members of the CIU and the necessary cooperation (the unions file strike notices).

First of all, it appears that most unions intend to keep control of the discourse on the hospital, for example, by provoking plethoric meetings with a multitude of union representatives: 'which led to meetings with 40 people at the AP-HP, which achieved nothing'.

The gap can be seen in the profile of those we call 'movement activists', an indigenous category used by radical political activists precisely to iden-tify 'new faces' in the movements. 'Very rich personalities, most of them first-time activists', 'rare union members', Hugo Huon summarises con-cerning the CIU. According to a later interview (Hugo Huon, 17 June 2021), the new activist had no militant experience and did five years of SAMU social, with an 'orientation towards vulnerable patients', as he says. He is 32 years old, with 7 years of seniority, 6 of which were in the emer-gency room. Before the CIU, he was accustomed to reading the *Canard Enchaîné* newspaper but was not a union member. His first intense 'politi-cal' discussions took place during the movement; they were less a sign of predisposition than of verbal confrontation with representatives of institu-tions unfavourable to the CIU's self-managed initiative.

He talks about his close collaborators who were first-time activists in the CIU. Bleuen, 31 years old, 5 years of seniority, played a leading role in Saint Antoine Hospital and was the victim of an attack (by a patient) at the origin of the movement. She joined the union late in life to protect herself but had no militant culture. Claire was 34 years old and had worked in the emergency room for 10 years. She experienced her first movement with the CIU. She is not a union member. The 'Annecy team' was young and dynamic, ready and able to go to Paris but without a militant past.

For all that, the new activist neither rejects nor hides 'the militant cul-ture', whose (rare) presence he appreciates, which helped him to find his way in the movement. There is indeed an interrelation between this cul-ture and spontaneity (Snow & Moss, 2014), as we have seen with nurses critical of the hierarchy, even if not all culture is 'movementist', nor all activism predisposed to the same 'career', even if the test of immobility makes people want to get away. Bleuen quickly faded away, the victim of depression. Huon is now in charge of a vaccination centre, without having climbed many rungs. The meticulous and painstaking construction of the network of striking emergency wards in the provinces relied on two resource contacts, Béatrice and Fabrice. Béatrice, 38 years old, spent 10 years in the emergency room. She has a master's degree, but after the movement found herself 'in difficulty in retraining'. Fabrice, from Nantes, 'is still very involved', frequents the Economistes Atterrés, with an oppositional FO pedigree (Lambertist). He works part-time in a PASS (health and social services centre), 'focused on vulnerable patients' too. Samira, from the CNT, is young and racialised, and also has a militant culture. She now works in addictology. Charles from Nantes, a nurse's aide, 55 years old, 25 years of seniority, close to the LFI party, died of cancer. Nadine from Bordeaux, 45 years old, 20 years of seniority in the hospital, has a political culture stemming from her previous socialisation in the CGT, but she is very critical of the union. She was 'pushed out' of the hospital and now works as a prison nurse.

So, the gap between the CIU and the 'trade union milieu', as distinct from the reference wage base (Sainsaulieu, 2014), does not lie in the political culture. If, on the movement side, militant culture serves in the short term, a certain horizontal diversification of activities, spontaneity does not provide the upward movement reserved for the apparatus. 'People are promoted in the union more due to seniority than merit. With a weak political culture'. It is the lack of stature in this milieu that has kept him away from trade unionism. The Sud trade union lent a room 'the first month', and Olivier Youinou, secretary of Sud-APHP, has a 'big militant pedigree', as well as remarkable human qualities, but 'not at all comparable to what we come across in the unions'.

The contrast between *homo mobilis* and *immobilis* can be seen in the methodology of action. Starting with the way of counting, of conducting the survey:

The people from the APHP mentioned a lack of 700 posts, based on the SAMU Urgences France reference system. However, the collective went beyond this claim by carrying out quantitative and qualitative work, starting from the field, work on staffing levels. That's what showed our legitimacy. That's how we started to distinguish ourselves from the unions.

This coordination work involves building a network. The unions do not use their own pre-existing network to serve the movement. On the contrary, the collective movement depends on its capacity to build the network, which it must develop piece by piece, via direct canvassing of the care teams. For Candice Lafarge, 'it's hours and hours on the phone'.

Although initially approached by the CIU, the unions saw this outsider as a rival. A competition set in, a struggle for 'representativeness' within the movement, between the collective movement and the unions. The collective movement scored points in the action:

> There was a demonstration on 6 June. It was an important move because we organised the demonstration in the name of the collective movement. And it was a success, we distinguished ourselves from the unions. They held a demonstration on the 11th which didn't go down too well. So now we're weighing in.

However, this competition is not only horizontal. It pits a group of young people against experienced permanent staff, backed by an apparatus and a leadership:

> Mind you, with the people at the base, in the unions, it goes very well. It's really at the level of the management that we find that things aren't going well.

The union leaderships are evolving in another sphere: 'FO was very hostile to the movement, the CGT has evolved a little in the movement. The UNSA and the CFDT, we didn't see them. But they were present at the Ségur'. Unlike the CIU, which was excluded from the negotiation space. The gap between the movement's activists and union representatives pits the field against representation, but also mobilisation work against demobilisation work.

> Personally, I'm also tired. [...] And then what disgusts me the most is the crab basket aspect, especially with the unions and the government. You hear: "you're very kind but I can't", "I have my own issues, and I want to be re-elected next year", from both the government and the union. And in fact their own interests take precedence over public health. It disgusts me.

The institutionalisation of trade unionism has gone through historical stages, at the end of which it appears ambivalent: on the one hand, an advocate for employees; on the other, a particular 'group style' (Eliasoph & Lichterman, 2003), defending its interests, partly autonomous from those of its constituents (Sainsaulieu, 2017). In other words, trade unionism is not immune from the dynamics of professionalisation that mark the socio-political field, but also from the older process of bureaucratisation, which impoverishes its human resources.

While trade unionism is well established in the public services, carers are poorly unionised and lack militancy (Sainsaulieu, 2008). This does not undermine the institutional weight of the union as a social partner. In a public establishment of respectable size, they 'don't touch the unions', 'the management never attacks unionised staff', believes Claire, a nurse (in Huon, 2020, op. cit., p. 226). In the eyes of employees in general, however, the union remains a moral force at the service of the workforce and an individual recourse against management in the event of a problem (Sainsaulieu, 2014). For all that, neither its internal weight nor its legitimacy is automatically translated into collective action, alongside the militants from a movement.

## BIBLIOGRAPHY

Abbott, A. (2003). Ecologies liées. A propos du système des professions. In P.-M. Menger (Ed.), *Les professions et leur sociologie*. Editions de la maison des sciences de l'homme.

Arborio, A. (2009). §3. Les aides-soignantes à l'hôpital. Délégation et professionnalisation autour du "sale boulot". In D. Demazière (Ed.), *Sociologie des groupes professionnels: Acquis récents et nouveaux défis* (pp. 51–61). La Découverte.

Corcuff, P. (2009). Frustrations Relatives. In O. Fillieule (Éd.), *Dictionnaire des mouvements sociaux* (pp. 242–248). Presses de Sciences Po. https://doi.org/10.3917/scpo.filli.2009.01.0242

Demazière, D. (Ed.). (2009). *Sociologie des groupes professionnels: Acquis récents et nouveaux défis*. La Découverte.

Divay, S. (2013). §13—Infirmière: une profession au large éventail de carrières… horizontales. In J.-P. Cadet (Ed.), *Les professions intermédiaires. Des métiers d'interface au coeur de l'entreprise* (pp. 195–202). Armand Colin.

Divay, S., & Girard, L. (2019). Eléments pour l'ébauche d'une socio-histoire du groupe professionnel infirmier. Un fil conducteur: la formation des infirmières et de leurs cheffes. *Recherche en soins infirmiers, 139*, 64–83.

Divay, S., & Vega, A. (2022). L'évolution des carrières infirmières: Une technique d'enrôlement dans l'hôpital de demain. communication au colloque *L'hôpital par en haut ou par en bas?* Pierru F. et Sainsaulieu I., Sénat, Paris, 28 février.

Eliasoph, N., & Lichterman, P. (2003). Culture in Interaction. *American Journal of Sociology, 108*(4), 735–794.

Fantasia, R., & Voss, K. (2003). *Des syndicats domestiqués.* Répression patronale et résistance syndicale aux États-Unis. Raisons d'agir.

Gheorghui, M., & Vega, A. (2019). Sociologie des professions de soins: le sens et la vocation plus que la productivité. *Compétence, 6/2019.*

Gourgues, G. (2017). Occuper son usine et produire: stratégie de lutte ou de survie: La fragile politisation des occupations de l'usine Lip (1973–1977). *Politix, 117,* 117–143. https://doi.org/10.3917/pox.117.0117

Huon, H. (2020). *Urgences* (p. 336). Albin Michel.

Linhart, D. (2015). *La comédie humaine du travail—De la déshumanisation taylorienne à la sur-humanisation managériale.* Editions Erès, Coll. Sociologie Clinique.

Pierru, F. (2022). 5. Le 'système de santé' français ou la réforme par la crise. In O. Giraud (Ed.), *Politiques sociales: l'état des savoirs* (pp. 79–96). La Découverte.

Ridel, D., & Sainsaulieu, I. (2021). Démobiliser les soignantes? Logiques spatiales, organisationnelles et institutionnelles à l'hôpital. *Espace et société, 183*(2), 51–66.

Sainsaulieu, I. (2003). *Le malaise des soignants. Le travail sous pression à l'hôpital.* L'Harmattan.

Sainsaulieu, I. (2008). Le syndicalisme à l'hôpital. Sociologie d'une insatisfaction. Dossier Syndicalisme et santé, *Les Tribunes de la santé,* n°18, 83–94.

Sainsaulieu, I. (2014). Retour sur la notion de 'base syndicale'. Le milieu de la CGT des banques en tensions. *L'Homme et la Société,* n°193–194, juin–décembre, 13–41.

Sainsaulieu, I. (2017). *Conflits et résistances au travail* (p. 150). SciencesPo Les Presses, coll. "Contester".

Sainsaulieu, I. (2020). Les Gilets jaunes, un peuple sans classes? Lectures critiques. *Revue française de science politique, 70,* 271–286.

Snow David, A., & Moss Dana, M. (2014). Protest on the Fly: Toward a Theory of Spontaneity in the Dynamics of Protest and Social Movements. *American Sociological Review, 79*(6), 1122–1143.

Vigna, X. (2021). *Histoire de la société française, 1968–1995.* La Découverte.

# CHAPTER 6

# Conclusion: What If the Hospitals Were Co-managed?

**Abstract** This last chapter draws on the potential for mobilisation of carers observed during the pandemic or the emergency room strike to look at sustainable solutions for the hospital. How can the power of professionals be increased and health care improved in the common interest? We know the bureaucratic and corporatist failings of hospital governance, but we also know how management control has deleterious effects. In the long term, we need to find a way of giving power back to carers while counterbalancing it with citizen control. The logic of representation is not enough, we also need direct consultations, in particular the possibility for professionals to submit their proposals for the public hospital to a popular referendum.

**Keywords** Hospital democracy • People power • Users counter-power

The hospital is traditionally defined as a professional bureaucracy, based on the consideration of a double administrative and medical rationality (Mintzberg, 1982). The concept of 'bureaucracy' also has a dual nature: a principle of rational ordering and a type of Weberian domination, heightened in this case by a persisting logic of profitability. Consequently, bureaucracy constitutes both a rational organisational framework and a burden for any healthcare dynamic. In this bureaucratic universe, the trade union institution does not function differently, it is not made for gliding

I. Sainsaulieu, *Care Staff Mobilisation in the Hospital*, https://doi.org/10.1007/978-981-19-9354-1_6

through a storm and serves collective mobilisation less than individual rights.

The contrast is strong with multifaceted healthcare mobilisation, in a consensus/protest continuum. It is reinforced by budgetary targeting of the public hospital wage bill, instead of the cost of liberal medicine and drugs. So, it is out of the question for caregivers to have more power.

In the wake of the pandemic, many candidates in the 2022 presidential elections took up the issue of the hospital by calling for more carers to be hired or seeking to restore the public services in general. However, not only does the leading candidate in the polls, Emmanuel Macron, not advocate these measures, but successive left-wing governments have introduced public expenditure controls since the turn to austerity in 1983 (Eloire, 2020).

The 'left hand' of the state, as the sociologist Pierre Bourdieu used to say, offers little guarantee in this respect, and many observers have concluded that the state is in league with the market, large private groups and capital accumulation (Dardot & Laval, 2009). With regard to the media, which have been spectacularly won over by capitalist concentration, some colleagues propose developing democratic control by journalists and citizens.

Although the public hospital is not private, it is not exempt from the trend to reduce public spending. In order to defend it, we cannot rely on representation or ignore the need for better control of public policies by the main people concerned: users and hospital staff.

## 6.1    Relying on the Initiative of Healthcare Providers

It should be noted first of all that doctors once had more power over public hospitals. Many doctors, often from the right, defended their fiefdoms and exercised mandarin authority over lowly care workers, before later converting to hospital management. There is no question of returning to this feudal and bourgeois control of doctors from good families.

Other reforms have at one time focused on improving the quality of care, by soliciting the participation of carers, particularly during the accreditation of hospitals. Thus, medical and paramedical protocols were developed by the professionals themselves to improve the quality of care.

The pandemic also provided an opportunity for carers to take charge in the departments affected: in both hospitals and care homes, managers gave them the initiative. But, if their participation was required in the emergency, a return to order followed instead of any reorganisation of work.

It was not the first time. Periods of crisis or health emergencies often create a call to action for groups of workers, who find themselves in the heat of the action. This is the case during storms, heatwaves and various epidemics, and was particularly true during the AIDS outbreak, a memorable period which left its mark on the infectious diseases departments as much as on the participants in the associative movements outside the hospital walls. Each time, and more regularly in the emergency room or operating theatre, a particularly egalitarian collaborative dynamic develops, because, when faced with the unknown, we are all equal and everyone is called upon in the same way, from the ordinary employee to the doctor: we need everyone's opinion.

These are what I have called consensual mobilisations because, although they have no protest motive, they still create an inclusive dynamic which temporarily subverts the official and symbolic hierarchical approaches, in other words established according to rank and diploma, or according to gender and social origin. But why refer to such exceptional situations, however recurrent they may be, when there are official representatives, elected by hospital staff in professional elections?

## 6.2   WEAKNESS OF THE UNIONS

The hospital civil service has joint administrative committees and technical committees. Both are consultative and based on consultation between staff and management representatives to deal either with the personal career advancement of staff (CAP) or collective organisational issues (CTE) and play, at best, a pedagogical role in social dialogue.

There is little sociological literature on the sectoral functioning of joint committees. However, because of their consultative nature, their impact on the daily life of hospitals is doubtful. And in fact, in the 500 interviews I have conducted with all the professions in the hospital, in the course of 8 surveys on labour relations in the departments, no one ever mentioned it. In the French labour world, the unionised community has most often been a world apart, a minority: traditionally, it is mainly the highly committed activists who make the link with the non-unionised staff.

In the hospital, care workers who vote in professional elections are not in the majority and are less unionised in percentage terms than non-health workers. This can be explained by a form of individualism on the one hand, and a strong bureaucracy on the other. There are undoubtedly vicious circles in which weariness, disengagement and bureaucracy are maintained. In any case, everyone, including the unions, agrees that union time is taken up by consultation structures. The accumulation of mandates is a sufficiently explicit factor, regretted by the unions themselves: activists accumulate delegation mandates, due to a lack of candidates or a desire to cut themselves off from the world of work.

The experience of social struggles can also be mentioned. Why, on the rare occasions when carers have gone on strike, have they felt the need to build ad hoc committees instead of simply following the representative unions? This has happened at least twice, in 1988–1989 with the setting up of coordination bodies during the nurses' strike and in 2019 when a national strike council was created during the emergencies strike.

Unions often claim to represent employees de facto without feeling the need to place themselves under their control when employees mobilise. They do not seek to create an egalitarian mobilisation, precisely of the type experienced by carers as a result of health crises or emergencies that shake their work. To enter the union structure, you often have to grasp the bureaucratic ethos, where concern for the structure comes before concern for the staff. But to work in a team, you have to be able to rely on others.

Activists, whether union members or not, have encountered the hostility of the federal apparatus during high-profile strikes. During the recent emergency room strike, the inter-emergency committee, an offshoot of the national strike council, asked for their help in vain and even felt hampered by the apparatus. So if neither the administration, nor the doctors, nor the trade union apparatuses can rely on the mobilisation of healthcare workers, then who can?

## 6.3    THE SOCIAL AND POLITICAL TABOO
### OF PEOPLE POWER

France is based on an elitist tradition, republican rather than democratic. National sovereignty has always prevailed over popular sovereignty, except in rare moments of revolutionary upsurge. The Rousseauist principle of the general will, which is the foundation of democracy and the general interest, has remained an empty word.

In view of the problems created by the current top-down model, and sharing the general interest concerns of health and health cost control, the legitimate question is to increase the power of carers in the hospital. They do not decide on anything, and it is hard to see how to improve the organisation of work without changing this state of affairs. If we are interested in improving the quality of care, making savings, retaining staff and recruiting and training new staff, then no one is better placed than the hospital staff themselves. Indeed, they know their business, and they are in touch with it, and that is why we rely on their initiative in difficult situations, such as during the recent pandemic.

Above all, what useless expenses does staff has usually in mind? A glossy communication plan? A big, expensive event? Bringing in expensive consultants? Selling expensive drugs? Wanting a clientelist 'public-private partnership'? Constructing a showcase building? Hiring staff with no useful link to the service? Even pay rises would not take on indecent proportions if the staff had their say. Especially not for the best-paid medical specialties! This is what interviews with carers suggest, but also historians and sociologists of the working classes, who highlight a specific 'moral economy' or popular habitus, which is known to be more collective or oriented towards the useful and necessary, due to their socialisation. In the hospital, the team spirit at work prolongs the modest income and sense of economy of the working classes.

The taboo comes from above, it is political and social. Indeed, if managerial reforms have nibbled away at the power of doctors, it has not been given to employees but led to the reduction of the only budgetary item where we think cuts can legitimately be made: the wage bill. So, the ONDAM shows the evolution of the savings made on the backs of hospitals and not on those of private medicine, not to mention the price of drugs imposed by the pharmaceutical industry. Yet not only could greater power for hospital staff lead to finding sources of savings elsewhere, at the expense of laboratories and private medicine, but above all they could better manage the wage bill, including their own.

Of course, any instituted power, however popular and broad it may be, has its limits. There is no doubt that greater power for staff would also generate blockages, routine and abuses, not because of its social nature but because of the nature of majority power: however democratic it may be, it can constrain a minority on the one hand, and on the other hand, it may not be interested in groups other than those it represents—such as, in this case, the users. So how can the risks of this new majority power be limited?

## 6.4   The Counter-power of Users

There is no doubt that counter-powers should be found here, particularly among hospital users. This is not a simple question, because hospital users are by definition irregular, except for the chronically ill. But there are groups, such as patient or neighbourhood associations, which can also have a say in hospital management. For the time being, user participation in bodies is sparse and under top-down control. For example, hospital boards include a few 'users' appointed by the Regional Health Agencies. This participation could be made more democratic, by ensuring that the most disadvantaged people are not the least involved.

Beyond that, it should be possible to consult the population on the major options, by means of a referendum. Political orientation should be subject to democratic control, instead of limiting democratic power to the choice of individuals.

We must reinvent a whole system of governance from below, which really is a 'revolution', to use the title of the book by candidate Emmanuel Macron, who was certainly thinking more of a neoliberal revolution to break free of the 'old world'. Let's say that this revolution would be rather neo-popular and neo-democratic, far from the bosses of the supposedly digital 'new economy' or the old one. Not 'whatever it takes', but rather to control the public costs of public spending. With sufficient means, but under careful control.

Rebalancing and restoring power from below is necessary but would not be enough. It would also be necessary to keep intact the strength of employee mobilisation and its capacity for initiative in response to events. The reactivity of carers in the face of illness should have its counterpart in the management of institutions, as these must be able to adapt to daily changes. So it would be necessary to invent forms of challenge to the institution, rotation and renewal of the people in charge, calls for voluntary work and above all for initiative. So that everyone can test out their intuition, and even the possibility for everyone to campaign, to freely submit a project to the votes of others. We must retain the creative power of the institution and its spontaneity linked to the event.

Obviously, such a democratic and movement-oriented philosophy is not limited to the healthcare sector—or even to journalists, as mentioned above. The Communards understood this well, as they laid down the principle of a whole democratic rethinking of power and work in 1871 (Marx, 1871). So why start with the hospital? Perhaps precisely because it shows us where the emergency lies.

## Bibliography

Dardot, P., & Laval, C. (2009). *La nouvelle raison du monde*. La Découverte.

Eloire, F. (2020). Le "tournant de la rigueur" comme processus régulatoire: Étude d'une décision de politique économique. *Revue française de sociologie, 61*, 207–241.

Marx, K. (1871). *The Civil War in France*. Brochure.

Mintzberg, H. (1982). *Structures et dynamiques d'organisation*. Editions d'organisation.

# BIBLIOGRAPHY

Abbott, A. (1988). *The System of Professions*. University of Chicago Press.

Abbott, A. (2003). Ecologies liées. A propos du système des professions. In P.-M. Menger (Ed.), *Les professions et leur sociologie*. Editions de la maison des sciences de l'homme.

Abecassis, P., Coutinet, N., Juven, P., & Vincent, F. (2019). La santé, un business? In: Fondation Copernic (Éd.), *Manuel indocile de sciences sociales: Pour des savoirs résistants* (pp. 142–150). La Découverte.

Andolfatto, D. (Dir.). (2007). *Les syndicats en France*. Paris: La Documentation Française.

Andolfatto, D., & Labbé, D. (2000). *Sociologie des syndicats*. Paris: La Découverte, Repères.

Arborio, A. (2009). §3. Les aides-soignantes à l'hôpital. Délégation et professionnalisation autour du "sale boulot". In D. Demazière (Ed.), *Sociologie des groupes professionnels: Acquis récents et nouveaux défis* (pp. 51–61). La Découverte.

Ariès, P. (1992). Adaptation aux temps nouveaux ou résurgence de tendances profondes: le Syndicat Général du Personnel des Hospices Civils de Lyon de 1939 à 1944. *Le Mouvement Social*, n°158, Le syndicalisme sous Vichy, 17–36.

Arnault, S., Fizzala, A., Leroux, I., & Lombardo, P. (n.d.). L'activité des établissements de santé en 2006 en hospitalisation complète et partielle. *Etudes et Résultats*, n°618.

Askenazy, P., Dormont, B., Geoffard, P., & Paris, V. (2013). Pour un système de santé plus efficace. *Notes du conseil d'analyse économique*, 8, 1–12.

I. Sainsaulieu, *Care Staff Mobilisation in the Hospital*, https://doi.org/10.1007/978-981-19-9354-1

87

Audric, S., & Niel, X. (2002). La mobilité des professionnels de santé salariés des hôpitaux publics. *Etudes et Résultats*. DREES.

Avril, C. (2009). Une mobilisation collective dans l'aide à domicile à la lumière des pratiques et des relations de travail. *Politix, 86*, 97–118.

Avril, C. (2018). 15—Sous le *care*, le travail des femmes de milieux populaires. Pour une critique empirique d'une notion à succès. In M. Maruani (Ed.), *Je travaille, donc je suis. Perspectives féministes* (pp. 205–216). La Découverte.

Avril, C., Cartier, M., & Serre, D. (2010). *Enquêter sur le travail: Concepts, méthodes, récits*. Paris: La Découverte.

Avril, C., & Ramos Vacca, I. (2020). Se salir les mains pour les autres. Métiers de femme et division morale du travail. *Travail, genre et sociétés, 43*, 85–102.

Baim-Lance, A., Tietz, D., Lever, H., Swart, M., & Agins, B. (2018). Everyday and Unavoidable Coproduction: Exploring Patient Participation in the Delivery of Healthcare Services. *Sociology, Health and Illness, 41*(1), 128–142. https://doi.org/10.1111/1467-9566.12801

Bajos, N., Spire, A., Silberzan, L., & for the EPICOV Study Group. (2022). The Social Specificities of Hostility Toward Vaccination against Covid-19 in France. *PLoS ONE, 17*(1), e0262192. https://doi.org/10.1371/journal.pone.0262192

Barozet, E., Sainsaulieu, I., Cortesero, R., & Mélo, D. (2022). *Where Has Social Justice Gone? From Equality to Experimentation*. Palgrave Macmillan.

Barreau, J. (Dir.). (2003). *Quelle démocratie sociale dans le monde du travail?* Presses universitaires de Rennes.

Benallah, S., & Domin, J.-P. (2017). Intensité et pénibilités du travail à l'hôpital. *Travail et Emploi* [En ligne], 152 | octobre–décembre, mis en ligne le 01 octobre 2019. http://journals.openedition.org/travailemploi/7755

Boltanski, L., & Thévenot, L. (1991). *De la justification. Les économies de la grandeur*. Gallimard.

Bourdieu, P. (2022). *L'intérêt au désintéressement. Cours au collège de France, 1987–1988*. Seuil.

Bourret, P. (2006). *Les cadres de santé à l'hôpital. Un travail de lien invisible*. Ed. Seli Arsan.

Branciard, A., Mosse, P., & Guegan, L. (1994). *Hôpital, Innovations, Professions*. LEST.

Canguilhem, G. (1972). *Le normal et le pathologique*. Presses Universitaires de France.

Castel, R. (1995). *Les métamorphoses de la question sociale* (p. 490). Une chronique du salariat. Fayard.

Castra, M., & Sainsaulieu, I. (2020). Intervenir sur un autre territoire professionnel. Equipes mobiles et services sédentaires à l'hôpital. *Sciences sociales et santé, 38*(4), 47–74.

Cazes, B. (1993). *Motsei Ostrogorski. La démocratie et les partis politiques.* In *Politique étrangère*, n°2, 58ᵉannée, 516–517.

CFTC, section CFTC des services de santé et services sociaux. (1985). 50 ans d'action syndicale en secteur sanitaire et social, Confédération Française des Travailleurs Chrétiens.

Chevandier, C. (2000). Connaître les militants hospitaliers des trois premiers quarts du XIXème siècle: analyse d'un corpus prosographique. *Journée d'étude sur le militantisme hospitalier.* Université Paris 1, Centre d'histoire sociale.

Cognet, M. (2020). Les services de santé: lieu d'un racisme méconnu. In O. Slaouti (Ed.), *Racismes de France* (pp. 74–86). La Découverte.

Corcuff, P. (2009). Frustrations Relatives. In O. Fillieule (Éd.), *Dictionnaire des mouvements sociaux* (pp. 242–248). Presses de Sciences Po. https://doi.org/10.3917/scpo.filli.2009.01.0242

Dall'Ora, C., Ball, J., Reinius, M., & Griffiths, P. (2020, June 5). Burnout in Nursing: A Theoretical Review. *Human Resource Health, 18*(1), 41.

Dardot, P., & Laval, C. (2009). *La nouvelle raison du monde.* La Découverte.

Demazière, D. (Ed.). (2009). *Sociologie des groupes professionnels: Acquis récents et nouveaux défis.* La Découverte.

De Troyer, M. (2001). Le secteur hospitalier en Europe. *Newsletter-BTS.*

Delaunay, J.-C., & Gadrey, J. (1987). *Les enjeux de la société de service.* Presses de Science Po.

Dhoquois, G. (1966). Le mode de production asiatique. *Cahiers Internationaux de Sociologie, 41,* 83–92. http://www.jstor.org/stable/40689370

Diallo, A. M., & Sainsaulieu, I. (2022). Les agents de « santé communautaire » au Sénégal. Unité et segmentation d'un groupe semi-professionnel en milieu rural et péri-urbain. *Sciences sociales et santé, 40,* 5–28.

Divay, S. (2013). §13—Infirmière: une profession au large éventail de carrières... horizontales. In J.-P. Cadet (Ed.), *Les professions intermédiaires. Des métiers d'interface au coeur de l'entreprise* (pp. 195–202). Armand Colin.

Divay, S., & Girard, L. (2019). Eléments pour l'ébauche d'une socio-histoire du groupe professionnel infirmier. Un fil conducteur: la formation des infirmières et de leurs cheffes. *Recherche en soins infirmiers, 139,* 64–83.

Divay, S., & Vega, A. (2022). L'évolution des carrières infirmières: Une technique d'enrôlement dans l'hôpital de demain. communication au colloque *L'hôpital par en haut ou par en bas?* Pierru F. et Sainsaulieu I., Sénat, Paris, 28 février.

Dorlin, E. (2017). *Se défendre. Une philosophie de la violence.* Zones éditions.

Dubost, Cl., Pollack, C., & Rey, S. (2020). Les inégalités sociales face à l'épidémie de Covid-19. *Les dossiers de la DREE*, n° 62.

Dubois, V., & Lieutaud, M. (2020). La 'fraude sociale' en questions. La naturalisation d'une thématique politique au prisme des questions à l'assemblée nationale (1986–2017). *Revue française de science politique, 70*(3–4), 341–371.

Eliasoph, N., & Lichterman, P. (2003). Culture in Interaction. *American Journal of Sociology, 108*(4), 735–794.

Eloire, F. (2020). Le "tournant de la rigueur" comme processus régulatoire: Étude d'une décision de politique économique. *Revue française de sociologie, 61*, 207–241.

Ernst, J. (2020). Professional Boundary Struggles in the Context of Healthcare Change: The Relational and Symbolic Constitution of Nursing Ethos in the Space of Possible Professionalisation. *Sociology, Health and Illness, 42*(7), 1727–1741. https://doi.org/10.1111/1467-9566.13161

Fantasia, R., & Voss, K. (2003). *Des syndicats domestiqués*. Répression patronale et résistance syndicale aux États-Unis. Raisons d'agir.

Ferguson, J., Tazzyman, A., Walshe, K., Bryce, M., Boyd, A., Archer, J., Price, T., & Tredinnick-Rowe, J. (2020). 'You're just a locum': Professional Identity and Temporary Workers in the Medical Profession. *Sociology, Health and Illness, 43*(1), 149–166. https://doi.org/10.1111/1467-9566.13210

Francfort, I., Osty, F., Sainsaulieu, R., & Uhalde, M. (1995). *Les mondes sociaux de l'entreprise*. Desclée de Brouwer.

Gaxie, D. (2005). Rétributions du militantisme et paradoxes de l'action collective. *Swiss Political Science Review, 11*(1), 157–188.

Gheorghui, M., & Vega, A. (2019). Sociologie des professions de soins: le sens et la vocation plus que la productivité. *Compétence, 6/2019*.

Gheorghiu, M. D., & Moatty, F. (2013). L'hôpital en mouvement. Changements organisationnels et conditions de travail: Rueil-Malmaison, éditions Liaisons, [Noisy-le-Grand], Centre d'études de l'emploi, coll. "Liaisons sociales".

Gilligan, C. (2009). Le care, éthique féminine ou éthique féministe? *Multitudes, 37–38*(2–3), 76–78.

Gilligan, C. (2019). *Une voix différente. La morale a-t-elle un sexe?* Champs-Essais.

Giraud, B. (2009). Des conflits du travail à la sociologie des mobilisations: les apports d'un décloisonnement empirique et théorique. *Politix, 86*, 13–29.

Glenn, E. N. (2000). Creating a Caring Society. *Contemporary Sociology, 29*, 84–94.

Gourgues, G. (2017). Occuper son usine et produire: stratégie de lutte ou de survie: La fragile politisation des occupations de l'usine Lip (1973–1977). *Politix, 117*, 117–143. https://doi.org/10.3917/pox.117.0117

Graeber, D. (2015). *Bureaucratie, l'utopie des règles*. Les liens qui libèrent.

Gurr, T. (1971). *Why Men Rebel?* Princeton University Press.

Guttierez-Crocco, F. (2012). Les archipels militants dans le syndicalisme chilien ou la frontière revisitée entre syndicalisme et politique. In I. Sainsaulieu & M. Surdez (Dir.), *Sens politiques du travail*. Armand Colin, coll. "Recherche".

Hassenteufel, P. (1991). Pratiques représentatives et constructions identitaires: une approche des coordinations. *Revue Française de Science Politique, 41*(1), 5–27.

Hibou, B. (2012). *La bureaucratisation du monde à l'ère néolibérale*. La Découverte.

Hill Collins, P. (2008). La construction sociale de la pensée féministe Noire. In E. Dorlin (Dir.), *Black Feminism, Anthologie du féminisme africain-américain, 1975–2000* (pp. 135–175). L'Harmattan.

Hocquelet, M. (2014). Les passés composés de la grande distribution: De l'appropriation managériale au support des contestations salariales. *Sociologies pratiques, 29*, 63–72.

Huon, H. (2020). *Urgences* (p. 336). Albin Michel.

Ibos, C., Damamme, A., Molinier, P., & Paperman, P. (2019). Le *care* justifie le sacrifice des femmes. Dans: Ibos, Damamme, Molinier, & Paperman (Dir.), *Vers une société du care. Une politique de l'attention.* Le Cavalier Bleu.

Jacoby, S. M. (2004). *Employing Bureaucracy.* Taylor & Francis Group.

Jacobzone, S. (2002). Les apports de l'économie industrielle pour définir la stratégie économique de l'hôpital public. DESE, INSEE.

Kelly, J. (1998). *Rethinking Industrial Relations. Mobilization, Collectivism and Long Waves.* Routledge.

Kentish-Barnes, N. (2007). Décisions de fin de vie en réanimation. *Revue Française de Sociologie, 48*(3), 449–475.

Kergoat, D. (1992). *Les infirmières et leur coordination, 1988–1989* (p. 192). Editions Lamarre.

Kergoat, D., Imbert, F., Le Doare, H., & Senotier, D. (1992). *Les infirmières et leur coordination.* Lamarre.

Lallement, M. (1996). *Sociologie des relations professionnelles.* La Découverte.

Lallement, M. (2007). *Le travail. Une sociologie contemporaine.* Gallimard.

Le Lan, R. (2006). La réduction du temps de travail vue par les salariés hospitaliers en 2003. *Etudes et résultats.* DREES, 03/469.

Le Lan, R., & Baubeau, D. (2004). Les conditions de travail perçues par les professionnels des établissements de santé. *Etudes et Résultats.* DREES.

Leicht, K. T., Walter, T., Sainsaulieu, I., & Davies, S. (2009). New Public Management and New Professionalism across Nations and Contexts. In New Governance and New Professionalism, n° spécial, *Current Sociology*, Sage, *57*(4), 581–605.

Lequeux, S., & Sainsaulieu, I. (2010). Social Movement Unionism in France: A Case for Revitalisation? *Labor Studies Journal, 35*(4), 503–519.

Linhart, D. (2015). *La comédie humaine du travail—De la déshumanisation taylorienne à la sur-humanisation managériale.* Editions Erès, Coll. Sociologie Clinique.

Lipszyc, B., & Laurent, S. (2000). L'absentéisme dans une institution hospitalière: les facteurs déterminants. *Cahiers économiques de Bruxelles, 166*(4), 131–170.

Lochard, Y., Meilland, C., & Mouna, V. (2006). *La tête de l'emploi. Discriminations raciales et marchés du travail: les salariés hautement qualifiés dans les télécommunications et à l'hôpital.* DARES/IRES.

Longchamp, P., Toffel, K., Bühlmann, F., & Tawfik, A. (2020). *L'espace infirmier. Visions et divisions d'une profession.* Livreo-Alphil, Neuchâtel, 258.

Marx, K. (1871). *The Civil War in France.* Brochure.

Marx, K. (1971). *La guerre civile en France*. Editions sociales.

Marx, K. (2014). *Le 18 Brumaire de Louis Napoléon Bonaparte*. Fayard/Mille et une nuits.

McAlevey, J. (2016). *No Shortcuts: Organizing for Power in the New Gilded Age*. Oxford University Press.

Michels, R. (2015). *Sociologie du parti dans la démocratie moderne. Enquête sur les tendances oligarchiques de la vie des groupes*. Gallimard, Folio Essais.

Mintzberg, H. (1982). *Structures et dynamiques d'organisation*. Editions d'organisation.

Molinier, P. (2005). Le care à l'épreuve du travail. Vulnérabilités croisées et savoir-faire discrets. In Le souci des autres. Ethique et politique du care, P. Paperman, & S. Laugier (Dir.), *Raisons Pratiques* (pp. 299–316). Editions de l'EHESS.

Moll, A., Moser, I., & Pols, J. (2010). *Care in Practice: On Tinkering in Clinics, Homes and Farms*. Transcript Verlag. https://doi.org/10.14361/transcript.9783839414477

Mouriaux, R. (2006). Syndicalisme et politique: liaison dangereuse ou tragédie moderne? *Mouvements, 43*(1), 30–35.

Nachtwey, O. (2020). *La société du déclassement. La contestation à l'ère de la modernité régressive*. Editions de la Maison des Sciences de l'Homme.

Nickelsen, M., & Niels, C. (2019). The Infrastructure of Telecare: Implications for Nursing Tasks and the Nurse-Doctor Relationship. *Sociology, Health and Illness, 41*(1), 67–80.

Nugus, P. (2019). Re-structuring the Negotiated Order of the Hospital. *Sociology, Health and Illness, 41*(2), 378–394. https://doi.org/10.1111/1467-9566.12838

Ostrogorski, M. (1912). *La démocratie et les partis politiques*. Calmann-Lévy.

Paperman, P., & Molinier, P. (2011). L'éthique du care comme pensée de l'égalité. *Travail, genre et sociétés*, 2011/2, n° 26, 89–193.

Parsons, S. (2021). Support Workers and the Health Professions in International Perspective. *The Invisible Providers of Health Care, Mike Saks, Bristol: Policy Press, Sociology, Health and Illness, 43*(7), 1720–1721. https://doi.org/10.1111/1467-9566.13303

Paugam, S. (2001). *Le salarié de la précarité*. Presses Universitaires de France.

People's Health Movement. (2021). *A Political Economy Analysis of the Impact of Covid-19 Pandemic on Health Workers*. Yale Law School.

Perrot, M. (1973). *Les Ouvriers en grève. France 1871–1890*. Mouton.

Picot, G. (2005). Entre médecins et personnel infirmier à l'hôpital public: un rapport social instable. Dynamiques professionnelles dans le champ de la santé. *Revue Française des Affaires Sociales*, n°1, Janvier–mars, 83–100.

Picot, G. (2008). L'encadrement au féminin: le rôle de l'interpersonnel. In I. Sainsaulieu (Dir.), *Les cadres hospitaliers. Représentations et pratiques*. Lamarre.

Pierru, F. (2022). 5. Le 'système de santé' français ou la réforme par la crise. In O. Giraud (Ed.), *Politiques sociales: l'état des savoirs* (pp. 79–96). La Découverte.

Pinell, P. (2009). La genèse du champ médical: le cas de la France (1795–1870). *Revue française de sociologie, 50*(2), 315–349.

Pouchelle, M.-C. (1998). Ici, on ne fait pas de cadeau. Partages du temps et don de soi à l'hôpital. *Ethnologie Française, XXVIII*(4), 540–550.

Raynaud, P. (1989). Société bureaucratique et totalitarisme. Remarques sur l'évolution du groupe 'Socialisme ou Barbarie'. In G. Busino (Ed.), *Autonomie et autotransformation de la société. La philosophie militante de Cornelius Castoriadis* (pp. 255–268). Librairie Droz.

Reich, A. D. (2012). *With God on Our Side: The Struggle for Workers' Rights in a Catholic Hospital*. Cornell University Press.

Ridel, D., & Sainsaulieu, I. (2021). Démobiliser les soignantes? Logiques spatiales, organisationnelles et institutionnelles à l'hôpital. *Espace et société, 183*(2), 51–66.

Rosanvallon, P. (1988). *La question syndicale*. Calmann-Lévy.

Sainsaulieu, I. (1999). Sud-PTT: A Political Trade Unionism? *Industrial Relations, 54*(4), 790–814.

Sainsaulieu, I. (2003). *Le malaise des soignants. Le travail sous pression à l'hôpital*. L'Harmattan.

Sainsaulieu, I. (2006). *La communauté de soins en question. Le travail hospitalier face aux enjeux de société*. Lamarre.

Sainsaulieu, I. (2007). *L'hôpital et ses acteurs. Appartenances et égalité*. Belin, Perspectives sociologiques.

Sainsaulieu, I. (2008a). Le syndicalisme à l'hôpital. Sociologie d'une insatisfaction. Dossier Syndicalisme et santé, *Les Tribunes de la santé*, n°18, 83–94.

Sainsaulieu, I. (2008b). Le cadre animateur: figure fragile d'une conciliation légitime. In I. Sainsaulieu (Dir.), *Les cadres hospitaliers. Représentations et pratiques*. Lamarre.

Sainsaulieu, I. (2009). Le bon patient est sous contrôle. Communautés de service et pratiques soignantes à l'hôpital. *Revue suisse de sociologie – Swiss Journal of Sociology, 35*(3), 551–570.

Sainsaulieu, I. (2012). Collective Mobilisation in Hospitals: Confrontational or Consensual? *Revue française de sociologie (English), 53*(3), 316–346.

Sainsaulieu, I. (2014). Retour sur la notion de 'base syndicale'. Le milieu de la CGT des banques en tensions. *L'Homme et la Société*, n°193–194, juin–décembre, 13–41.

Sainsaulieu, I. (2017). *Conflits et résistances au travail* (p. 150). SciencesPo Les Presses, coll. "Contester".

Sainsaulieu, I. (2020). Les Gilets jaunes, un peuple sans classes? Lectures critiques. *Revue française de science politique, 70*, 271–286.

Sainsaulieu, I. (2021a). Mobilisations soignantes par gros temps: quelle prise de risque organisationnelle? Point de vue, *Revue française des affaires sociales*, n°4, 97–109.

Sainsaulieu, I. (2021b). Over-mobilisation, Poor Integration of Care Groups: The French Hospital System in the Face of the Pandemic. *Forum for Social Economics, 13*(1), 207–219.

Sainsaulieu, I., & Saint-Martin, A. (Eds.). (2019). *L'innovation en eaux troubles. Sciences, techniques, idéologies* (p. 329). Editions du Croquant.

Sainsaulieu, I., & Vega, A. (2014). Introduction. *Les Sciences de l'éducation—Pour l'Ère nouvelle, 47*(3), 7–11.

Salaun, F. (2000). La problématique syndicat-association professionnelle aux sources du syndicalisme hospitalier. *Journée d'étude sur le militantisme hospitalier*. Université Paris 1, Centre d'histoire sociale.

Scambler, G. (2018). *Sociology, Health, and the Fractured Society: A Critical Realist Account* (p. 208). Routledge.

Simonet, M. (2018). *Travail gratuit, la nouvelle exploitation*. Editions Textuel.

Siwek-Pouydesseau, J. (1989). *Les syndicats de fonctionnaires depuis 1948*. Presses Universitaires de France.

Siwek-Pouydesseau, J. (1996). *Le syndicalisme des cols blancs*. L'Harmattan.

Smith, H. L. (1970). Un double système d'autorité: le dilemme de l'hôpital. In C. Herzlich (coord.), *Médecine, maladie et société* (pp. 259–262). Ecole pratique des hautes études/Mouton.

Snow David, A., & Moss Dana, M. (2014). Protest on the Fly: Toward a Theory of Spontaneity in the Dynamics of Protest and Social Movements. *American Sociological Review, 79*(6), 1122–1143.

Strauss, A. (1992). *La trame de la négotiation*. L'Harmattan.

Surdez, M., Zufferey, E., Sainsaulieu, I., Plomb, F., & Poglia Mileti, F. (2018). *L'enracinement professionnel des opinions politiques. Enquête auprès d'agriculteurs, d'ingénieurs et de directeurs de ressources humaines exerçant en Suisse*. Seismo.

Tackett, T. (1997). *Par la volonté du peuple. Comment les députés de 1789 sont devenus révolutionnaires*. Albin Michel.

Tronto, J. (2009). *Un monde vulnérable, pour une politique du care* (*Moral Boundaries: A Political Argument for an Ethic of Care*, 1993). La Découverte.

Trotsky, L. (1940). *Les syndicats à l'époque de la décadence impérialiste*. Brochure.

Vega, A. (2000a). L'apolitisme infirmier. Journée d'étude sur le militantisme hospitalier, Université Paris 1, Centre d'histoire sociale.

Vega, A. (2000b). *Une ethnologue à l'hôpital*. Editions des Archives Contemporaines.

Vigna, X. (2021). *Histoire de la société française, 1968–1995*. La Découverte.

Vincent, C., & Volovitch, P. (2002). *Les syndicats face aux restructurations hospitalières: entre défense des personnels et gestion des systèmes de santé*. Institut de Recherche et d'Etudes sur le Syndicalisme.

Visier, L. (1992). L'image des syndicats dans les gros établissements hospitaliers. Confédération Française Démocratique du Travail.

Voisin, C., & Faugere, J.-P. (1981). *Les emplois hospitaliers. Une approche économique*. Economica.

Printed in the United States
by Baker & Taylor Publisher Services